Mare Island
Naval Hospital

Mare Island Naval Hospital

A History, 1864–1957

Thomas L. Snyder, M.D.

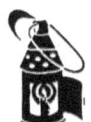

McFarland & Company, Inc., Publishers
Jefferson, North Carolina

ISBN (print) 978-1-4766-9738-3
ISBN (ebook) 978-1-4766-5526-0

Library of Congress cataloging data are available

© 2025 Thomas L. Snyder. All rights reserved

No part of this book may be reproduced or transmitted in any form or by any means, electronic or mechanical, including photocopying or recording, or by any information storage and retrieval system, without permission in writing from the publisher.

Front cover images: Photograph of Main Hospital Building, Mare Island, California. U.S. Naval Hospital, 1925 (Naval History and Heritage Command); *insets, left to right*: Spraying sailors' throats with carbolic acid, photograph by Ammen Farenholt, 1918 (National Archives, Washington, D.C.); Captain Henry Howard Kessler (left) and LCDR Douglas D. Toffelmier observe a sailor's new Mare Island prosthetic, official Navy photograph, Mare Island Historic Park Foundation, Vallejo, California.

Printed in the United States of America

McFarland & Company, Inc., Publishers
Box 611, Jefferson, North Carolina 28640
www.mcfarlandpub.com

This book is dedicated to the memory of Professor Harold D. Langley, who became a friend and mentor as I embarked on my "second career" as a historian of maritime medicine. Harry was a pioneer in the field, having published the first history of American naval medicine—*A History of Medicine in the Early U.S. Navy* (Johns Hopkins University Press, 1995)—and was an early supporter of my effort to establish the Society for the History of Navy Medicine in 2008.

An emeritus professor of history at the Catholic University of America in Washington, D.C., and curator of the Smithsonian's Naval Collection, Harry was a very proper historian: he always dressed in tie and jacket, even when he was plumbing the depths of the National Archives (where younger researchers often show up in T-shirts and flip-flops).

And he was a wonderful, encouraging teacher, advising me to avoid being distracted from my primary historical goal (this book) by the multitude of historical rabbit holes I'd find as I did my research. (He was right. I was indeed distracted—this project has taken 20 years to complete!) I wrote this dedication while Harry was still alive, so he knew my intent and my devotion to him and to his memory.

Table of Contents

Preface	1
Introduction	5

Part I—The Early Years: Anticipating Modern Health Care

One. The Navy Arrives on the West Coast	15
Two. Early Medical Care at Mare Island Navy Yard	18
Three. A Firm Base for Health Care and the Doctors	29
Four. A Hospital in Technological Transformation, 1871–1898	42
Five. Early 20th Century	85
Six. Toward Modernity	97

Part II—The 20th Century: Responding to World Events

Seven. First "Test of War"	125
Eight. Interbellum	132
Nine. Into the Great Depression and Then Ramping Up	142
Ten. World War II—Their Finest Hour	149
Eleven. War's End, Immobilization, Korean War, Closure	163
Epilogue	175
Chapter Notes	179
Bibliography	203
Index	207

Preface

I began my undergraduate education as a history major but soon found the reading burden to be far too great for my short attention span. Biology and physics were much easier, and I ended up with a bachelor of arts in chemistry—an ideal (at the time) "pre-med" degree. Then followed medical studies in Albany, New York, and residency in Chicago (interrupted by three years' active Navy duty in destroyers plying the South China Sea, and at the Naval Postgraduate School in Monterey, California). I practiced urology with the Kaiser-Permanente Health Care Program in Northern California and served as "twice a citizen"[1] in the U.S. Navy Reserve.

While "distracted" by my profession and life in general, I nevertheless retained my love for history. So it was natural that when I retired from the Navy Reserve (1987) and from my practice (2003), I should combine my naval and medical interests to research and write the history of the Navy's first West Coast hospital, which just happens to be located in the (now former) Navy Yard on Mare Island, directly across the Napa River from my hometown of Vallejo, California.

What followed was ten years of quarterly trips to the National Archives in Washington, D.C., and College Park, Maryland, where the archivists—bless them!—have retained correspondence between hospital commanders and the officials at the Navy's Bureau of Medicine and Surgery. Side trips to the National Archives in San Bruno, California, and to the History Office of the Navy Bureau of Medicine and Surgery supplemented my research. The 100-year-old correspondence at first consisted of letters on stout paper, handwritten and copied no doubt by yeomen (but signed by the originator—I touched

Preface

Farragut's[2] signature several times over the course of my archival work), with pages often stuck together, having been wetted by some unknown person and requiring the most delicate separation of pages. Next came tissue paper copies: the tissue paper was dampened, placed on the original to soak up enough of the ink to provide very crisp and readable renditions of the originals. Finally, somewhere around 1895, typewritten and then carbon copies became standard. When handwritten, the letters were concise, using words economically but exceedingly well. With the advent of the typewriter, readability increased a lot (even yeomen sometimes had writing that was difficult to decipher), but so did the number of words! The quality of the writing, however, most definitely did not improve.

This correspondence very nicely carried the historical narrative until about 1930, when the volume of letters suddenly dropped off. This, I think, is due to the telephone. Now, instead of writing or telegraphing higher headquarters, the hospital commander could simply pick up the phone and call in his request for guidance. It's then that I began to depend on the local Vallejo press and, later, official Mare Island newspapers to carry the narrative.

As my research progressed, three historical "themes" began to suggest themselves. They are the intrepidity of the men (and, later, the women) who labored to serve the sailors, Marines and civilian workers here in the frontier; a spirit of creativity and resourcefulness from the earliest days; and, later, a theory about medical architecture. You will see them expressed from time to time as you read.

Throughout the volume, you'll see extensive quotes from the correspondents—the true narrators of the story. These quotes are essential to give you a sense of the times and environments in which they worked and the ways they thought about their work.

The "template" for this volume is the slide presentation, variations of which I've given to numerous academic and civic organizations over these several years to tell the story of the naval hospital at Mare Island. Touro University California now owns the hospital campus. Medical students and others now walk the hallowed ground where heroes once trod.

Preface

Finally, a historical work, no matter its length or depth, is really a work of many people. Archivists at the National Archives in Washington, D.C.—as well as in College Park, Maryland, and San Bruno, California—are famous and respected for their work in preserving our national heritage and making it pretty readily available for researchers like me. André Sobocinski, historian, and Michael Rhode, archivist, at the Historical Office of the Navy Bureau of Medicine and Surgery offered assistance and invaluable advice at many stops in the 20-plus years this work has taken up. Thanks also to the collection of local newspapers residing in the basement of the Vallejo Naval and Historical Museum, and the terrific photo collection in the library of the Mare Island Historic Park Foundation on the old Navy Yard itself. A dear Navy friend and colleague, Captain Odette Willis, NC, USN (Ret.), was the hotelier and dinner chef for nearly all of my quarterly 2-week research visits to the DC area. Words of thanks do not suffice...

My most important collaborator and guide has been my wife of more than 50 years, Gina. To her wisdom and support I owe almost every success I've enjoyed in life. She did it with loving, persistent support that became more like urging as both the project and I wore on, ending in the past few years with "If you don't finish your book before you die, I will kill you!" Thank you, my love!

(A note on abbreviations: You will see the term "BuMed" [pronounced "byoo med"] frequently in this book. It stands for "Bureau of Medicine and Surgery," the administrative center for all Navy and Marine Corps medical activities. The Navy has a long tradition of truncated abbreviations and acronyms—there's even a publication, known colloquially as "NavDic,"[3] that offers a comprehensive listing—because it historically operated under what we today would refer to as "narrow bandwidth" conditions—communication by flags, semaphores and signal lights. Imagine a string of "letter" flags spelling out the entire "Bureau of Medicine and..."; there wouldn't be a yardarm long enough or ship's mast tall enough. Hence, "BuMed.")

Introduction

In the West, mention of physicians serving aboard naval vessels goes back to the Greek poet Homer, who, in the *Iliad*, has the naval leader Machaon bring his family tradition of healing to the successful treatment of arrow-wounded King Menelaus. The Roman navy is believed to have paid its surgeons double the army rate (*duplicarii*) to encourage their service in the less prestigious—and riskier—military arm. During the late Middle Ages, the Italian maritime republics routinely posted surgeons[1] aboard ships, and during the Crusades, naval surgeons established shore-based facilities for the care of injured and sick sailors. Medical officers of Genoa and Venice were responsible for issuing health certificates to sailors of these navies; these officers also established port quarantine (from Italian *quarantina giorni*—"40 days") procedures for prevention of imported contagion, especially the plague.

In the modern era, the Spanish and French were early to adopt standing naval medical establishments, maintaining naval hospitals in colonial territories. While the British Royal Navy had surgeons aboard ships from the 15th century, they did not form what might be recognized as a formal medical corps until 1805, when, for the first time, surgeons of the Royal Navy were granted rank similar to other military officers and a distinguishing uniform. The earliest American Continental Navy Regulations from 1775 implied the presence of surgeons aboard our men-of-war. The ships' captains hired them, typically for the duration of a single cruise or mission. The Naval Act of 1794—taken as the official establishing document of our Navy—specified that the president of the United States would

Introduction

"commission" surgeons but as "civil officers" without military rank. Military "equivalent" ranking (ranging from "assistant surgeon" to "passed assistant surgeon" to "surgeon") came in 1841. Additional ranks of "medical inspector" and "medical director" were added in 1871. Navy General Order No. 418 of August 15, 1918, instituted the ranks we use today—the same Ensign through Rear Admiral as used for "line" officers[2] but with the sobriquet "Medical Corps" added.

While places for the care of the poor and travelers (care of the sick usually being provided in their homes) are described in early Chinese and Indian literature, it appears that these facilities were "ad hoc" enterprises, often set up in the homes or on the grounds of local leaders or wealthy men but not as permanent establishments organized on the basis of any public policy. The history of hospitals, as we understand the term, has its beginning with the Roman army. As the empire grew geographically, it became increasingly difficult (and costly) to transport ill or injured soldiers back to their homes in Italy for care. Moreover, well-trained legionnaires were too valuable to send home if they could be cured where they were stationed on the frontiers of the empire. Thus evolved, around 100 BCE, the Roman *valetudinaria*—facilities, both permanent and "mobile," that had many of the attributes we associate with modern hospitals—individual rooms with beds, galleys for food preparation, pharmacies for preparation of medications, and accommodation for assigned military surgeons (*milites medici*) and their assistants (*capsarii*, named for the bandage box—*capsa*—they carried).[3] Some of the larger facilities have been found to contain sophisticated kits of surgical instruments.

This concept of the hospital seems never to have found its way into the civilian realm in Roman times. It was the early Christians, motivated by Christ's evocation of care and compassion for the poor, who offered the first hints of what would become hospitals in the West. These were originally found mostly in the eastern part of the Christian realm (Constantinople). Called *xenodochia*, they were really places for the general accommodation of travelers and the poor, with no intention for the treatment of the ill. From the

Introduction

fourth century CE, monasteries, which spread extensively throughout Europe and Britain, commonly provided accommodation for visitors and travelers, and they usually had small separate facilities for the care and healing of their monks (who, as an educated class, often also developed medical expertise). However, only rarely was this care offered, as a matter of policy, to the lay population.[4] As the Roman imperial governance in Europe waned, church governance—local bishops—replaced it. Basil, bishop of Caesarea, established what is probably the first civil hospital in the West, in 389 CE. Up through the 11th century, a few urban hospitals, usually sponsored by local bishops or wealthy donors, sprung up. Dominated by church doctrine and dogma, these facilities offered charity care, any medical treatment being limited to a healthy-diet-and-liturgy regimen.

While medical doctrine and treatment languished in the medieval West, hospital development and medical studies flourished during the "golden age of Islam" in the ninth to 13th centuries. The caliphs of Baghdad sponsored an extensive translation program that brought classical ancient Greek medical texts to the Arab world. In addition, following the Qur'anic imperative to care for the sick, the caliphs established a network of sophisticated hospitals, called *bimaristans* (from Persian "bimar"—sick person or patient—and "stan"—place or location). These institutions were unique in that they provided free care to the needy and the traveler. They featured specialty clinics (including surgery), had in-house pharmacies and frequently offered teaching programs for aspiring physicians. Their operation was typically financed by income from properties given to them by wealthy patrons.[5]

The "hospital movement" in the West gained momentum as a result of a crude cross-fertilization of ideas arising from the Crusades, where Europeans first came into contact with (and sometimes received care in) *bimaristans*.[6] The prototype of Western hospitals seems to be one that was originally organized around 1080 in Jerusalem, by Amalfi merchants, for the accommodation of pilgrims and merchants. Later operated by the Order of St. John (later known as

Introduction

the Knights Hospitaler because of their support of the hospital) incident to the first and subsequent Crusades, the enterprise expanded its care to soldiers and the sick. The Hospitalers expanded into a few European cities, and as pilgrims and crusaders returned home, they brought the hospital idea with them, causing the movement to spread throughout the Christian realm. By the late Middle Ages and into the Renaissance, the hospital movement spread. The combined effects of the Reformation and humanism reduced the church's influence but broadened the support of hospitals to include civic governments. In addition, hospitals became increasingly "medicalized"[7]—that is, the emphasis on care shifted from care of the soul to care of the body, with increasingly scientific medical principles applied. Stimulated by a release from church dogma and restrictions on scientific study, by the 15th century, famous medical universities emerged, first in Italy, then in Paris and in larger cities throughout Europe.

An early "prototype" naval hospital—for the care of old and destitute sailors—was established in Venice in 1318. To the French goes credit for the first hospital specifically designated as "naval"—*Rochefort*—constructed around 1666, incident to the creation of Louis XIV's navy.[8] The British established a retirement hospital for Royal Navy seamen at Greenwich in 1588. A tax on the pay of each sailor supported the hospital. In 1729, the tax was extended to sailors from the American colonies, though few actually ended up at Greenwich since they preferred to receive care nearer home.[9]

In the colonies, the maritime community of Virginia addressed the matter by setting up a sailors' hospital in Norfolk in 1758. The Virginia government itself authorized a sick and disabled sailor hospital in 1780, paid for by a tax on the sailors' pay. Work on the hospital finished in 1789. It took a naval war—the police actions against the Barbary States—to prompt the creation of a temporary American naval hospital, in a Sicilian house large enough to accommodate 100 patients, in 1804. The cessation of the police action against Tripoli in 1805 eliminated the need for the hospital, and it closed in early 1806.[10] From around the time of the War of 1812, the Navy

Introduction

leased homes near shipyards in Brooklyn, Philadelphia, Washington and New Orleans to serve as hospitals. In Boston (Charlestown), part of the marine barracks filled the need. Although Congress discussed and debated establishment of permanent naval hospitals as early as 1810, it wasn't until 1828 that Congress actually appropriated money for this. The first purpose-built U.S. Naval Hospital opened in Norfolk, Virginia, in 1830.[11]

The practice of medicine and surgery in the mid–19th century was beginning to emerge from the centuries-long influence of Galenism, which held that disease was the result of imbalances between four "humors"—black bile, yellow bile, blood and phlegm. In this system, doctors sought to right the imbalances by such interventions as bleeding (often two or more pints at a sitting), emetics (inducing vomiting) and purgation (inducing bowel evacuation). Because the causes of disease were still not understood, medicines were often given to treat symptoms only. For instance, cinchona bark, the source of quinine, was prescribed for any high fever (based solely on its beneficial effect on the fevers of malaria for which quinine was add then an effective cure). Whereas contagion was understood, its causes were not. For instance, much emphasis was placed on bad air ("mal'aria," in Italian) as a cause of disease. Accordingly, great emphasis was placed on finding locations on high ground, offering breezes of clean air, for hospital placement. The performance of surgery was emerging as a result of the development of effective anesthesia, but it was still fraught because the cause of infection had not yet been elucidated. Once the bacterial theory of infection had been established, however, surgery became safer, though still looked upon as a "last resort" undertaking. Because medical education in the United States was often a catch-as-catch-can proposition, starting in 1828, the Navy required all physicians desiring a commission to have a medical degree and to pass a rigorous oral examination of their knowledge of anatomy, chemistry, materia medica, medical jurisprudence and obstetrics.

Introduction

A Note About Mare Island

Mare Island, California, the "home" of this narrative, is really a peninsula that lies along the west side of the Napa River as it enters the north end of San Francisco Bay. Local legend, reported as fact by Arnold Lott, author of the 1954 official history of the Navy Yard,[12] has it that the "island" received its name when the Mexican governor of California, General Mariano Guadalupe Vallejo, saw his favorite white mare—which he thought had drowned when the barge on which she was being transported on the Napa River capsized—happily grazing on that flat land. So pleased was he to see the horse alive and well that he was moved to name the land on which she was roaming "Isla de la Yegua," which translates less poetically as "Mare Island."

The Navy Yard that Commander David Farragut established on the island (see below) was the Navy's first on the West Coast. Naval activity started slowly there, with the arrival of a floating drydock, transported in sections around the Cape of Good Hope and reassembled in the Napa River, adjacent to the Navy Yard. It took five years before Mare Island produced its first ship, USS *Saginaw*, launched in 1859. By the time America entered World War I, the shipyard's workforce had expanded to around 10,000 skilled craftsmen. Those workers still hold the record for the fastest destroyer built in the United States—the USS *Ward* (DD-139)—just 17½ days from keel laying to launch in 1918.

After a lull during the Great Depression, navy yard activity picked up in anticipation of the coming conflict. At its World War II peak, nearly 50,000 men and women—the largest workforce in California at the time—worked 24/7 to build and repair ships and submarines for the war effort. According to Arnold Lott, the 22 submarines built at Mare Island during the war were responsible for sinking 252 enemy ships—988,357 tons.[13]

After the war, the Navy called on Mare Island's skilled men and women to build nuclear submarines, starting in 1957 with the USS *Sargo* (SSN 583) and ending in 1970 with USS *Drum* (SSN-677).

Introduction

Submarine repairs and nuclear refueling continued until 1995. The shipyard closed in 1997, a victim of the end-of-the-20th-century Base Realignment and Closure process.[14]

Part I

The Early Years
Anticipating Modern Health Care

ONE

The Navy Arrives on the West Coast

From their founding, the 13 United States did not have a naval presence in the Pacific Ocean, even as East Coast commercial and whaling traffic in those faraway waters increased. Naval elements of the world's oceanic hegemon, Britain, were not averse to stopping American-owned ships and pressing those deemed as his majesty's subjects into their own crews. Shipwrecked American sailors had no one to look to for their rescue, and there was no American presence to ensure that American commercial and maritime laws were being enforced. And then there were the Sandwich Islands (Hawaii)—a tropical paradise with huge commercial potential—that the Royal Navy was sniffing around. Finally, there was no naval force present to represent American interests in working out the northwestern border between the United States and Canada.

This all changed in 1821, when the U.S. Pacific Squadron was stood up. Usually made up of five ships and based in Valparaiso, Chile, and Callao (Lima), Peru, elements of the squadron ranged out into the Pacific as far as the Chinese coast (while keeping a naval eye on Hawaii) and as far north as the 49th Parallel, where the United States and Britain finally agreed to set the border in 1846.[1]

As unseemly as it might appear, a North American anchorage for the squadron was impossible so long as the Pacific Coast was in Mexican hands. American concerns about British designs on the west coast of North America led to a preemptive naval takeover of the capital of Mexican California, Monterey, in October 1842. Upon discovery that the United States and Mexico were not at

Part I—The Early Years

war (communications were slow in those days before the telegraph or radio), this somewhat precipitous act was immediately reversed. However, the deed had been done, and the Naval officer responsible, Thomas ap Catesby Jones, was recalled to Washington, D.C., and temporarily banished to command of the receiving ship[2] in New York Harbor.

But American interest in California and the Pacific was just beginning. That same year, Navy Secretary Abel Upshur, estimating the value of American whaling activity at $40 million, advocated for a large increase in the Pacific squadron to protect American Pacific commerce and to provide Americans living in an unstable Mexican California the "protection of our naval power."[3]

Four years later, the United States was in fact at war with Mexico, and while most of the wartime activity took place on the southern border of Texas, Commodore John D. Sloat repeated the act of the aggressive young Catesby Jones and once again occupied Monterey and San Francisco from the sea. This time, the takeover "stuck." There would be no return of California to Mexican control. The war with Mexico ended with the Treaty of Guadalupe Hidalgo (1848), in which Mexico ceded to the United States a huge swathe of land that included the present states of California, Nevada, Utah and New Mexico and larger or smaller portions of Arizona, Colorado, Oklahoma, Kansas and Wyoming. Almost simultaneous with the treaty, gold was discovered in California. This brought a huge migration of fortune seekers and the commerce necessary for their support, and before long the population of the heretofore sparsely populated area was large enough to qualify for statehood. Seeking effective civil government to keep order, Californians pressed vigorously for statehood, requesting admission as a "free state"—that is, one where slavery would be prohibited. Seven months of debate in the Senate ended with the Compromise of 1850—actually five statutes, one of which was the admission of California. Navy Secretary William Graham wrote to President Fillmore that "a new empire has, as by magic, sprung into existence. San Francisco promises, at no distant time, to become another New York." He concluded, "A navy yard is

One. The Navy Arrives on the West Coast

very much needed in California, and no time will be lost in accomplishing the work."[4] Navy Secretary Gideon Welles had already sent a commission of officers to scout out possible anchorage sites in 1848, and Graham followed up with another in 1852. This latter group, led by Commodore Sloat, directed its entire attention to the San Francisco Bay. Washington authorities apparently weren't interested in Southern California, perhaps because of its distance from the newly established U.S.-Canada border. Sloat's team spent several weeks surveying the bay and ultimately decided that Mare Island, 30 miles distant from the Golden Gate and therefore somewhat protected from possible Royal Navy predations, would be the ideal anchorage site. Once negotiations with a few squatters on the island were completed, it was duly purchased, and in 1852, a floating drydock constructed in New York and transported in pieces around Cape Horn was reassembled in the Napa River, next to Mare Island, across the river from the city of Vallejo, then the capital of the state of California. A couple of years later, on September 14, 1854, Commander David Farragut[5] arrived with his family. After settling his wife and son temporarily in the only house on Isla de la Yequa, he officially took possession and command of Mare Island two days later.[6]

Two

Early Medical Care at Mare Island Navy Yard

In nearby Sausalito was moored the second-class sloop-of-war USS *Warren*,[1] then serving as a receiving ship. Under orders from the new Commandant, she was towed the short trip east across San Francisco Bay and arrived at Mare Island on the 18th. Upon her arrival, the American flag flew over Mare Island shipyard for the first time. Though a small vessel, she counted among her crew Assistant Surgeon John Mills Browne, who would be the first Navy Medical Officer to set foot on the new Navy Yard. *Warren* served as the yard's first "hospital." Browne, an 1852 graduate of the Harvard Medical Department, had joined the Navy fresh out of medical school.[2] Now here he was, a lone Medical Officer on the Pacific frontier—no Stanford down the road to which to send his complicated cases. Browne's tenure was short—he departed in May 1855, but he returned later to play an important role in the medical history of the yard. We will see him several times in this story. He will end up as the Surgeon General of the Navy.

Assistant Surgeon Browne held "sick call" in *Warren*, and patients requiring hospital care would be lodged in wooden bed frames suspended from the ship's sick bay overhead or in their own hammocks. An idea of the Medical Officer's workload can be gleaned from Surgeon B. Reusch Mitchell's "Statistics of Quarter December 31st 1855":

Remaining from Sept 30	8 patients
Admitted during quarter	41 patients
Total no. under treatment	49 patients

Two. Early Medical Care at Mare Island Navy Yard

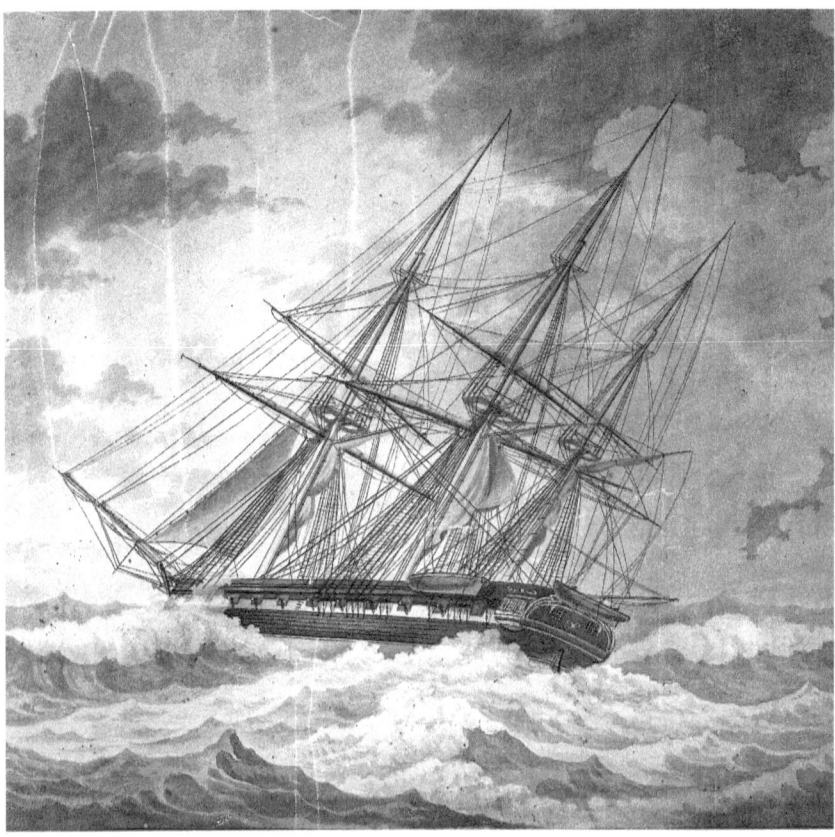

Sloop of War *Warren*. Detail from *U.S. Sloop Warren—1848* by Joseph Partridge (1947.0849.000004). Courtesy Mariners' Museum, Newport News, Virginia.

Discharged from list	45 patients
Remaining today	4 patients
Whole no. of rations	1,356
Daily average no. sick	$14^{738}/_{1,000}$
Daily average cost per man	3 cents 8 mills & $^{1}/_{10}$

Health care was a bargain back in the day!

Farragut very early recognized the unsuitability of ships as hospitals. In a June 15, 1855, letter to the Secretary of the Navy, he noted, "I shall propose to the Bureau, so soon as the Store House is finished, to appropriate the present temp^y Store House as a Hospital, as we feel the necessity of one daily" and, in October, forwarded his Civil Engineer D. Turner's "rough estimate of the cost of building.... Temporary Hospital: $5000."[3]

The new yard surgeon B. Reusch Mitchell wrote along the same lines, suggesting the conversion of the little receiving ship *Warren* into a hospital. Medicine and Surgery Bureau Chief William Whelan seemed to agree with the need for a hospital but not with Mitchell's USS *Warren* conversion idea. To Mitchell he wrote, "I doubt much if it be the purpose of the [Navy] Department that the '*Warren*' be converted into a Hospital Ship for the various vessels serving on the Pacific Station; I shall ask the attention of the Department to this part of your communication and invite some regulation on the subject." On the same day, November 14, 1855, he wrote to Secretary of the Navy James Dobbin, "The size of the squadron employed in the Pacific Ocean, and the advancing condition of the Navy Yard at Mare's [sic] Island renders a district Hospital Establishment highly necessary."

Space aboard the little second-class sloop-of-war (just 697 tons; 127' in length and with a beam [width] of only 33'9") must have been cramped under the best of circumstances. However, her role as receiving ship required her Medical Department not only to care for patients but also to be the medical storage and supply facility for the Navy Yard. The limitations of this arrangement prompted Surgeon John S. Messersmith in January 1857 to write to the Bureau of Medicine and Surgery, "I regret we have not a place better adapted for the storage of Medicines than the spirit room[4] of the *Warren*. Its narrow limits however are less objectionable than the constant humidity which pervades it and necessarily at an early day must prove injurious to them."[5]

The space situation improved somewhat with the arrival of the USS *Independence*, which became the yard's "hospital" in October 1857. Originally commissioned as a 90-gun ship of the line in 1832, the ship had been cut down—"razed"—by one deck to a 54-gun frigate. Now the fastest and most powerful ship in the Navy,

Two. Early Medical Care at Mare Island Navy Yard

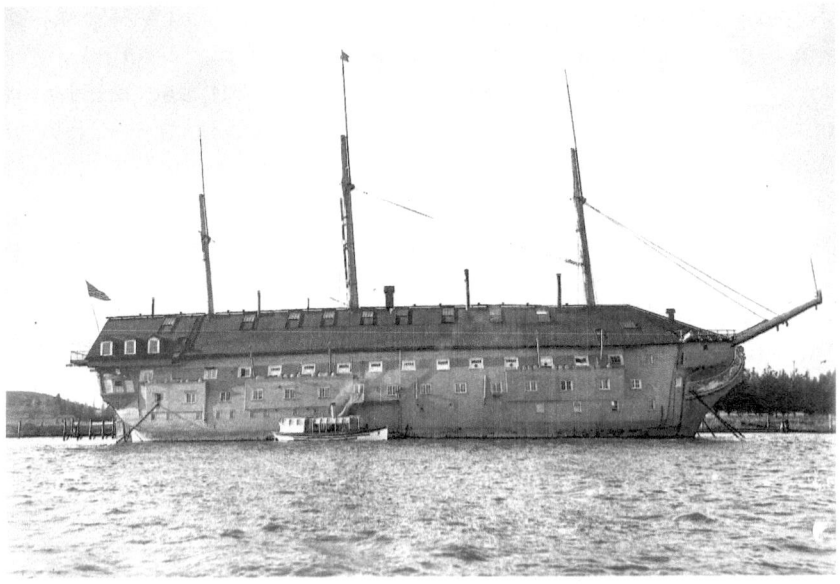

USS *Independence* as receiving ship, Mare Island Naval Ship Yard (date unknown). U.S. Navy Photo. Mare Island Historic Park Foundation, Vallejo, California.

Independence went on to have a distinguished career. The ship saw combat in the Mexican-American War in 1846 and served another ten years before becoming the Navy Yard's receiving ship. Even though substantially larger than *Warren*, the ship was still unsatisfactory as a medical care facility. Surgeon William S. Bishop wrote the Bureau of Medicine and Surgery in 1863, "Particularly in the winter season [*Independence*] is a very unsuitable place to treat the sick. It is cold, wet, and open to every wind that blows."

Perhaps distracted by a much larger undertaking than a little Navy Yard in faraway California—the Civil War—Navy authorities failed to move on the matter. So the yard surgeon, Bishop, submitted a proposal to convert an unused granary for hospital use. Writing on April 1, 1863, Bishop sent the bureau "a proposition that I have made [to the Commandant of the Yard] with plans and estimated cost, that will give us accommodation for twenty beds, and in an emergency, by using the chapel, we could put up thirty beds."[6] His

Part I—The Early Years

drawings provided for a 25' × 25' first-floor ward and a 24' × 40'9" ward space above and called for a large cistern for year-round water supply,[7] an attached bath (approached from outside) and, nearby, an outdoor privy (you get some idea here of why we refer to the Navy of those days as made up of "men of steel and ships of wood"). I will deal with the water issue later in this book.

The bureau resisted the proposal. Replying to Bishop, BuMed Chief Whelan wrote,

"I have to acknowledge the receipt of your communication of the 16th ultimo with plan of proposed modifications of a portion of a public building in the Navy Yard Mare Island California to adapt it to Hospital use for the increased naval establishment at that post." He continued, not encouragingly,

> I shall make application to the Treasury Department, as has been done in other instances for the admission of Naval patients into the Marine [now Public Health Service] Hospital San Francisco, paying out of the hospital fund,[8] to the collector of the port the same rates of maintenance and treatment as it costs the government to support the sick from the Merchant Service. [This "application" was duly written on May 18, 1863.]

Director Whelan went on,

> Recently, at Newport Rhode Island where a number of persons connected to the Naval Academy has greatly increased, I observed very comfortable accommodation for sick officers aboard the *Constitution* [then the receiving ship at Newport]. A frame building was erected on the spar deck between the Fore and Main Mast, occupying most of the fore and aft space; it was elevated, say a foot above the deck, well lighted, ventilated and indeed in every respect it was quite as desirable as the hospital quarters on shore. I have conferred with the Chief of the Bureau of Construction on this point and he will give authority for the erection of such a building on the deck of the "Independence," if it meet your views. The roof can be made waterproof; glazed moveable windows will afford light and air. The galley of the ship might be used for kitchen purposes, and economy be subserved in other ways.

He closed on this more hopeful note: "You will observe that an appropriation of $25,000 has already been made [on March 3, 1863] for commencing a Hospital at Mare Island; after the arrangements are begun, it is presumed no time will be lost in its completion, that can be reasonably avoided."[9]

Two. Early Medical Care at Mare Island Navy Yard

But the men on the West Coast continued their campaign for a temporary hospital at Mare Island. On June 8, Yard Commandant Captain Thomas Oliver Selfridge, apparently unhappy with the pace of progress on his hospital, wrote to the Bureau of Yards and Docks:

> The great length of time that will elapse[10] before the Naval Hospital authorized ... will be in condition to receive patients, induces me to suggest the substitution of some building capable of accommodating fifteen or twenty patients for a temporary hospital. There is a wooden building in the yard, formerly the old storehouse, one and a half stories high measuring 30 by 23 which at very moderate expense could be converted to this use as it will require but little else besides partitioning off outhouses and a fence thrown around it. This house has been used as a granary near the stables, but ... it is altogether too large for this purpose.

He finished his letter by taking a shot at the notion of hospitalizing sailors in the 25-mile-distant San Francisco Marine Hospital: "The seamen of the Pacific Squadron have been admitted into the Marine Hospital at San Francisco, but they have universally, for some reasons unexplained, been very much disaffected."[11]

Surgeon Bishop addressed the notion of constructing the temporary hospital in *Independence*, writing to Director Whelan on July 1,

> I would have been very glad to have adopted your suggestion as to setting up temporary hospital accommodations upon the Independence, but it would have to interfere with other uses to which Major Garland [commanding the Marine Battalion] applies the spar deck as to seriously inconvenience him in his command. It is not only for the Marine battalion that hospital accommodation is needed at this station, but for the use of the vessels of the [Pacific] squadron.[12]

He enclosed and endorsed a letter from a colleague, Surgeon Harlan of USS *Saranac*, who wrote, in part,

> A better shelter is needed [for the patients] than a ship off San Francisco, where gusts of cold wind make every invalid shudder. If you can have a hospital or an apartment suited to protect these sufferers, I beg you to present the case to the Commodore of the yard, so that the men can be immediately sent up.[13]

Admiral Smith of the Bureau of Yards and Docks replied on July 6, "You can at your discretion prepare the building you refer to as a temporary hospital"[14] and indicated in a letter of August 13 that

Part I—The Early Years

"fitting up temporary Hospital will be charged to Hospital fund and to be refunded after your estimates and appropriations are made for next [fiscal] year."[15]

It is now apparent that two bureaus—Yards and Docks and Medicine and Surgery—were working at cross-purposes because on July 15, Surgeon Whelan informed Yard Surgeon Bishop that "the arrangements made with the Collector of the Port for the admission of Naval patients into the Marine Hospital at San Francisco will afford ample accommodation for most of those for whom removal from ship board is considered necessary." Dr. Whelan followed up with a letter to Commandant Selfridge along the same vein on August 5:

> Touching the want of accommodation for Officers, I am of the opinion it might be better in many respects to admit Officers likely to require Hospital treatment, and especially if protracted, into the Marine Hospital in San Francisco, according to the arrangement long since entered into with the Treasury Department.[16] This hospital is supposed to possess every advantage of construction, convenience, etc., and to be under the direction of a professional man of excellence.

Nevertheless, work on the temporary hospital moved briskly along, with Surgeon Bishop reporting on October 19 that "the Commandant is converting an old Granary by removal and repair into a temporary Hospital." Ten days later, he wrote that the temporary facility would be "ready for use six weeks or two months from this time."[17]

In November, Commandant Selfridge reported that he expected the facility to be ready for use "for all the patients of the Pacific Squadron—sometime in January," and he submitted an estimated cost of $3,977.50, with a 25 percent surcharge "to meet the probable discount on 'legal tender notes,'[18] bringing the total cost to $4971.87½."[19]

Indeed, the facility *was* ready for occupancy in January 1864— just shy of ten years after Farragut's first arrival on the West Coast. Surgeon Bishop wrote to the Bureau on January 6 that "the arrival of two cases from the USS *Jamestown* in the East Indies has determined Captain Selfridge to give me an order to procure the necessary

Two. Early Medical Care at Mare Island Navy Yard

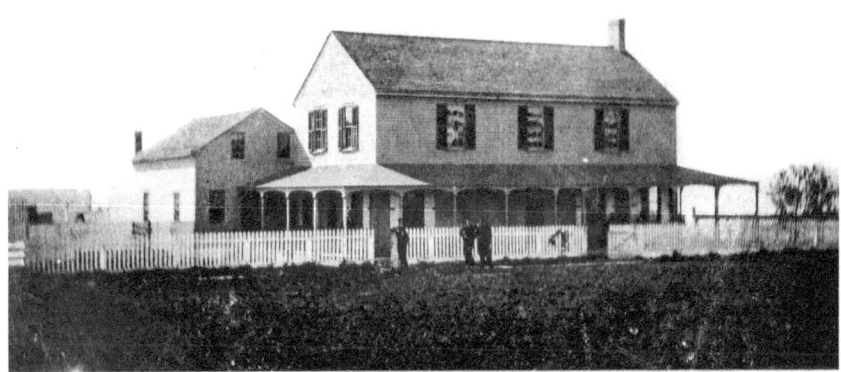

Granary as hospital on Mare Island. U.S. Navy Photo. Mare Island Historic Park Foundation, Vallejo, California.

appliances to receive patients in the temporary Hospital." He added that "though the Commandant's plan of constructing the temporary Hospital was not the one that I would have adopted, he has succeeded in making a very convenient place for twenty or thirty patients. I will commence moving the Dispensary and storeroom to the new building this week."[20]

Although never officially recognized as a hospital by the Navy Surgeon General, the facility carried an average inpatient load of 30 patients, cared for by a surgeon and a surgeon's steward. Not only did surgeons care for "medical" issues, but they performed surgery as well. For instance, in July 1871, Surgeon Bishop sent a special report back to Washington about a sailor who had been shot during a cutting-out expedition[21] off the Mexican coast, a musket ball having lodged in his left hip. Having no X-ray in that time, the surgeons probed the wound through the hole created by the projectile and estimated that the several fragments of bone would never heal. In constant pain, the patient was losing weight and clearly would die if something weren't done. Bishop recommended an operation to remove the shattered hip bones. He reported that the patient, upon "the nature of the case &c having

Part I—The Early Years

been explained to him ... cheerfully agree[d] to submit to anything that might be considered necessary." The surgery, performed by a team of eight doctors[22] under chloroform anesthesia, was a success. The patient, relieved of pain, began to gain weight, and after a period of rehabilitation, actually walked out of the hospital, fitted with an apparatus to support the limb that now lacked a hip joint.[23]

Recall that Congress, in March 1863, had passed an appropriation "For a Hospital, Mare Island, Cal of $25,000." Soon thereafter, BuMed Chief William Whelan requested Mare Island Navy Yard Commandant Thomas Selfridge to submit a site for the permanent facility. Selfridge very promptly appointed a panel of experts for this specific task, and on July 1, 1863, forwarded the panel's "report of a site for a Naval Hospital with a plan of the Yard showing the relative location" to the Bureau of Yards and Docks with an attached large chart of the island, with "Proposed site for Hospital" and "Hospital site as per App^d Plan" drawn and labeled. The proposed site appears to be close to the geographic center of the island. A penciled comment on the address side of Selfridge's cover letter, signed and dated (July 2, 1863) by civil engineer W.P. Sanger,[24] states,

> The reasons assigned by the Board for the selection made seem good and I recommend that the site proposed be adopted. When the original plan was made, no very particular attention was paid to the location of the Hospital, it not being considered properly as a Yard improvement; the site was marked, merely to show that a Hospital was thought of, and that there was ample room for it on the Island.

Selfridge's board of experts consisted of Surgeon Wm. Johnson, Jr.; Passed Assistant Surgeon Wm. S. Bishop; Assistant Surgeon W.C. Lyman; and Civil Engineer C. Brown. Their report listed several factors important in their selection of the site:

> 1st—its accessibility from the waterfront, and from the working portion of the Yard.
> 2nd—its sheltered position from the strong prevailing coast winds being directly under the lee of the high hills in its [illegible], giving it the advantage of the best aspects to the sun and an equality of warmth at all seasons.

Two. Early Medical Care at Mare Island Navy Yard

> 3rd—its relation to the best soil that the Island furnishes for gardens, and grounds, so essential to the comfort and economy of the institution.

On August 25, Selfridge received the bureau's reply, dated July 27, approving the hospital site.

Whelan wrote to Yard Medical Officer Passed Assistant Surgeon William S. Bishop on September 19, 1863. His concern was about the permanent hospital for which Congress had appropriated the funds:

> I beg to make some inquiries of you, as a professional man, in reference to the Hospital in progress at Mare Island, California. I may premise the remark that I am entirely ignorant of the location of the building, nor have I been consulted in regard its capacity, or internal arrangements.
>
> Hospital architecture, I need not observe, has become almost a specialty; it embraces ideas and adaptations outside the general scope of the profession [of architecture]..., and is never successful unless persons familiar with the peculiar province of a hospital [are involved with the design process].

Whelan went on to write a laundry list of concerns, ranging from soil characteristics to proper sewage to the orientation of the proposed building to the prevailing wind. He suggested the new Free City Hospital of Boston as the very model of a modern hospital, consisting of "a central, and detached buildings, connected by corridors which may be opened or closed, as appropriate.... This plan admits of ready extension, as necessity requires, and on the other hand, avoids the immediate construction of a building larger than ever be needed."[25] He complained that the $25,000 hospital appropriation had already "been expended in the preparation of the site, for the building." He closed with a request for the "joint opinions" of any Navy Medical Officers present on Mare Island and adjoining ships on all the matters raised. (I was unable to find any such survey.)

In May, the Surgeon General wrote to Selfridge to report that Congress had finally appropriated an additional $75,000 for the hospital. Added to the unspent portion of the earlier appropriation, he estimated that about $90,000 would be available to build the facility, which, to save costs, should be "a perfectly plain brick building of not exceeding 2 stories in height." By his specification of brick construction, it's clear that Director Whelan was not familiar with California earthquakes. Selfridge replied, "In the present depressed state of the currency, it would be inappropriate to build the new Hospital.... No one, I am confidant [sic], would offer to construct the entire building for the sum allotted in currency at the present time." Whelan concurred, "We shall let things remain as they are, till some more auspicious time presents for undertaking the work."[26]

The surgeons continued to provide medical and surgical care in the makeshift "temp[y] hospital" until Bureau Chief Horowitz contracted with Philadelphia architect John McArthur, Jr., to create a purpose-built hospital for the sailors and workers in this distant Navy Base.

THREE

A Firm Base for Health Care and the Doctors

On September 16, 1864, the shipyard's new Commandant, Captain D.W. McDougal, wrote to the new Director of the bureau, Dr. Phineas T. Horwitz, "I would call your attention to the limited accommodations for the sick at the present Hospital and recommend that work on the proposed Hospital be commenced at once." Horwitz, a month later, replied, "I beg to say, the [Navy] Department does not deem expedient to commence the erection of the N[ew] Hospital Building at Mare Island Cal at this time." Surgeon John M. Browne returned to Mare Island in April 1865, and he added his voice to the small chorus of complaint from California.

John McArthur, Jr., Philadelphia architect, was constructing the new naval hospital in his city when BuMed Director Horwitz first raised the notion of designs for the Mare Island project, writing (presumably in follow-up to verbal communication) early in June 1866 to acknowledge receipt of "sketches for California Hospital."[1] Two weeks later, he demurred, writing that "the unexpected rise in the premium on gold, will necessarily delay the commencement of the erection of the Naval Hospital at Mare Island."[2]

But the die was cast. Seemingly ready to commit to the project in July 1867, Horwitz wrote McArthur, "I will thank you to state what you will charge to furnish necessary drawing, working plans, and specifications of the building and appendages, complete"[3] and a week later telegraphed, "How long would you require to finish plans for Mare Island Hospital?"[4]

Four days later, Horwitz wrote to Mare Island Commandant

Part I—The Early Years

Thomas T. Craven, "I transmit the tracings for a Naval hospital to be erected at the Navy Yard, Mare Island, at the site selected" and requested that "the Civil Engineer of the Yard ... execute the necessary plans ... as it is intended by the Department to commence the erection of the Building as soon as possible after the examination and approval of the designs called for." He went on, "It may save time, and in a manner be a guide to the Department, in adding to, or reducing the proposed plan, if an approximative estimate of its cost can be ascertained from some of the most reliable builders in your vicinity."[5]

Director Horwitz appears to have been giving a double message, indicating to the people in California that things were to move along smartly, yet indicating to MacArthur that the weak dollar would cause a delay. Perhaps he was simply trying to keep the Californians "off his back" while he maneuvered the straits of political Washington, D.C.

It seems likely that his demand for formal drawings from the Mare Island Civil Engineer was just a clever delaying tactic, for it was a year later, on 29 October 1868 that Horwitz wrote in the Fiscal Year 1869–70 Naval Estimates: Mare Island Cal.—The Civil Engineer who was instructed to execute the necessary plans, elevations and specifications and materials and workmanship for erecting a hospital at this place, after consuming eleven months in carrying out the directions of the department, submitted estimates so far in excess of the appropriations of Congress, that it was found necessary to employ a professional architect to furnish all the designs and working plans, with printed descriptions and specifications. Mr Jno McArthur Jr has been selected for the purpose. His work will soon be completed when measures will at once be taken to commence the erection of the building.[6]

A month earlier, Horwitz sent McArthur a formal request for working drawings, noting that "the entire cost of the establishment, ready for occupation, including grading, cisterns, etc., etc. is not to exceed the amount appropriated by Congress for the purpose, viz. One Hundred Twenty Thousand dollars ($120,000)."[7] His "kicker": "It is to be understood that if the offer of the lowest possible bidder exceeds the amount appropriated by Congress, you are to receive no compensation for your services."

Three. A Firm Base for Health Care and the Doctors

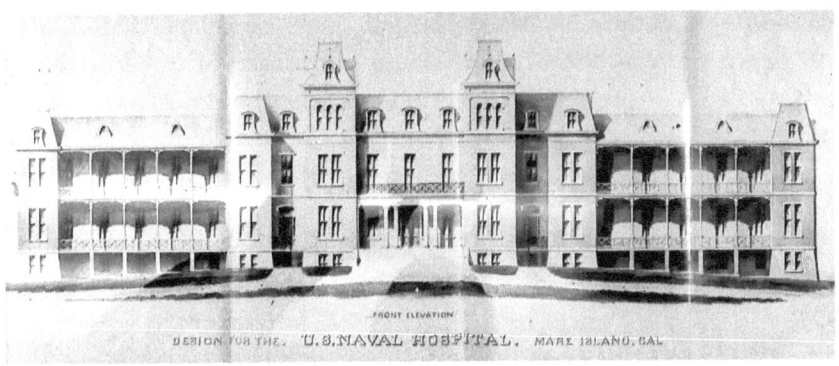

Architect John McArthur's cover illustration for plans of Naval Hospital, Mare Island, California, 1870. National Archives, Washington, D.C.

McArthur accepted the tough terms, with a fee of 3 percent of the accepted bid.[8] By late January 1869, he could report that the plans were "ready for the Photographer," and on February 9, he wrote to Dr. Horwitz at the bureau that "all the drawings and specifications for the contemplated Naval Hospital at Mare Island California have been forwarded to your office on this day."[9]

On January 18, Horwitz wrote to Dr. Browne,

> The Plans and Specifications for erecting a Naval Hospital at Mare Island, Cal., having been completed and approved, have been forwarded to the Commandant of the Naval Station at that place. [The records indicate the plans actually went into the mail on February 13. See below.] "Presuming that an offer to undertake the work within the amount appropriated by Congress will be received and accepted, you have been designated in conjunction with the Civil Engineer or other competent mechanic attached to the Navy Yard, to superintend the erection of the buildings. After the award has been made and the work begun, you will, with the engineer or other person selected to act with you as Superintendent, make monthly reports to the Bureau of the progress of the work."[10]

In his instructions concerning the letting of the construction contract, Horwitz was explicit: "It will be well for you to let it be understood that no bid will be considered which is in excess of the amount of the appropriation for the building of the hospital, viz., One hundred and twenty thousand dollars ($120,000) in currency" (Horwitz's underlining). As if for emphasis, he added, "Your attention is

Part I—The Early Years

called to the act of Congress of July 25, 1868, directing that no officer of the Government shall knowingly contract for the erection of any public building which shall bind the Government to pay a larger amount that the specified sum appropriated for such purpose."[11]

Acting Commandant Werden telegraphed receipt of the plans and instructions on March 19, indicating prompt compliance,[12] and on April 10, he forwarded copies of the advertisements for proposals for the new hospital to San Francisco's daily newspaper *Daily Alta California*.

Once again, however, the devalued currency caused problems, as Commandant Craven telegrammed the bureau on May 7, "Bid for Hospital two hundred and sixty four thousand dollars ($264,000). Would advise advertisement to build center and north wing which will serve at present. Can probably be done" and on May 11, "Offer to build center and one wing of hospital—one hundred and three thousand ($103,000) <u>coin</u>" (emphasis mine. Given a 25 percent adjustment for legal tender, this would amount to $128,750 in legal tender; building even half a hospital would exceed the congressional appropriation!).

Commandant Craven alluded to further correspondence on the matter in his telegram of June 18:

> In acknowledging the receipt of your letter of May 28th expressing the wishes of the Bureau in regard to the Hospital, I have to report that the contract for its erection was duly drawn up and signed on 8th inst [June]. As you were advised by telegram of 31st ult [May] Dennis Jordan—the lowest bidder—had offered to complete the building in eight months from the date of signing the contract.

Noting that with the onset of the California rainy season in but three months, he had "taken the responsibility" to extend the permitted construction period to one year.[13]

On June 25, Craven forwarded the complete list of bidders:[14]

Name	Address	Amt Asked	Time Required to Complete
S. Powell	Vallejo	$204,000	12 months from date of contract
D. Jordan	San Francisco	$148,000	8 months from date of contract
Geo. D. Nagle	San Francisco	$195,000	12 months from date of contract

Three. A Firm Base for Health Care and the Doctors

Name	Address	Amt Asked	Time Required to Complete
Chas H. Shaw	San Francisco	$150,000	No time specified
Chas Murphy	Vallejo	$169,000	No time specified
E.M. Benjamin	Vallejo	$178,000	12 months
David Akers	Vallejo	$185,000	12 months

Clearly, Dennis Jordan was paying close attention to his competition since he "came in" at just $2,000 below his nearest (San Francisco) competitor.

In a June 3 letter to the architect, Horwitz wrote, "The price of labor and materials having greatly advanced since the estimates of Civil Engineer Jno D Hoffman was [sic] submitted to the Bureau of Yards and Docks, upon which your calculations for building the Naval Hospital, Mare Island, Cal., were based, it has been found impossible to procure an offer to build the Establishment for the price named in my communication of Sept 21 ultimo." He went on to say that the contract had been signed and that the bureau would not hold McArthur to the "you won't get paid if the building cost exceeds $120,000" stipulation and paid him his fee of 3 percent—on $148,000.[15]

Charles Murphy of Vallejo received the contract for the hospital cistern—the water supply—at a bid of $7,633.

Work started immediately, with Dr. Browne and civil engineer Calvin Brown reporting on August 2 that necessary excavations were completed and that nearly 3,500 (cubic) yards of the removed earth had been used to construct a road across the tule[16] to "a small wharf, lately built, … sufficient for the reception and conveyance of all building material."[17]

On September 2, the bureau acknowledged receipt of the first contractor's bill—$11,200—for work performed from June 9 to August 14.

The Problem of Earthquakes—and a Solution (?)

Soon after construction began, Browne wrote the bureau that "with a view of strengthening the work as a precaution against earthquake effects, we recommend the introduction of a proper iron band in the brick work, as is generally being adopted in this vicinity."[18] Browne and his colleague, civil engineer Calvin Brown, estimated a cost of $1,000. On August 12, the civil engineer wrote,

> In obedience to your order of 11th inst [we] have enquired into the expediency of the introduction of an iron band into the masonry of the new Naval hospital now in progress on this Island, and are of the opinion that as recent experience of Earthquakes in this country demonstrates the necessity of guarding against their effects as far as possible, in brick buildings especially, by the introduction of a more continuous bond in the walls than is afforded by the ordinary manner of construction, which relies solely on the breaking of joints and the tenacity of mortar in which the bricks are laid, all buildings of this character should have their iron bars of suitable width laid between the courses of masonry at proper intervals, wherever the same can be carried continuously around the building unbroken by openings. Also, ... rods of iron should be carried up vertically as was done in the case of the Foundry chimney built in this Yard in 1862.[19]

He went on to describe how the foundry structure had survived the two heaviest earthquakes in the region while unreinforced chimneys had suffered major damage. Brown indicated that such reinforcements were standard practice in brick buildings being built in San Francisco and offered the opinion that their use was "indispensable." He recommended "not less than ten courses" of no. 15 American gauge[20] iron,[21] one and a half inches wide, be used in the walls and that vertical iron rods, one and one-fourth inches diameter, be introduced at the corners of the walls. Horwitz's assistant, Tryon, replied, sending a copy of recommendations from a local (D.C.) board of experts, which had the bureau's approval.

On October 12, Browne and Brown reported that they had "caused the Contractor to introduce an iron band" into the construction "in conformity with the instructions of the Bureau." Two additional circumferential bands (total of 12) were used. The total cost was $1,266 in currency.

Local Bricks—An "Experiment" That Made the Contract a Success

> I've noted that contractor Dennis Jordan came carefully in as the lowest bidder. I believe the reason he could do this was that he realized that brick for

Three. A Firm Base for Health Care and the Doctors

construction could be made on-site, thereby avoiding the cost of purchase and transport. On 2 August Browne wrote that the first kiln, "of 340,000 brick," had been fired, and noted that the clay was obtained in close proximity to the excavation for the Hospital.[22] On 6 September the Doctor and Engineer commented further:

> The brick, taken from the first kiln, situate at the edge of the excavation, are hard, of good color and of superior quality. It is gratifying that this experiment of brick making from Island clay is so decidedly a success. Mr Denio, Foreman Mason of the Navy Yard, asserts that these bricks are equal to any ordinary hard brick obtained by purchase.... A second kiln, of larger size, will be fired in a few days.[23]

On October 12, they reported, "The second kiln of brick in its entirety is equal to the first, and certain portions are superior, being in color, hardness and finish to be approximative to pressed brick. These will be employed in the exterior surface of the outer walls."[24] And on November 9: "The third and last kiln of brick has been burnt, supposed to be sufficient for the completion of the remaining brick work."[25] LCDR Arnold S. Lott, in his history of the Navy Yard, states that all together, one and a half million bricks were made on-site.[26]

In their final report, the superintendents wrote to

> commend the enterprise of the Contractor, Mr Jordan, in his experiment of making brick from clay at the site of the building. The result is a success, and demonstrates the feasibility of future manufacture of brick, of quality and quantity, to meet the requirement of the Department at this Navy yard.[27]

By early December 1869, the second-story walls were erected, and the south-wing roof was completed (important, for the Northern California rainy season is usually well along in December; apparently, the builders had so far enjoyed favorable weather). Gas pipes for lighting were being introduced "into several apartments in the south wing."[28]

A Couple of Significant Odds and Ends— Construction Progresses Nicely

In January 1870, Browne wrote,

> In reference to the supply pipes to the rain water cistern to the new Naval Hospital, it is provided in the specifications that they shall be of "terra cotta,

vitrified or cement pipes," put together with hydraulic cement. We are of the opinion that this material is not best adapted to conditions of the building and the locality of the cistern, and we would propose the substitution of iron pipes for the following reason. A portion of these pipes is laid beneath the basement floor which, in case of any derangement, would have to be taken up in order to get at and repair the damage. Pipes named in the specification are by no means strong, and the slightest shocks of an earthquake are sufficient to break them. In addition ... they cannot be made satisfactorily secure from leaks.... In dry country like this, it is of the utmost importance that every drop of water should be saved for use, and we believe that iron alone should be used for a conduit where this result is desirable.[29]

Permission for this change was immediately granted.[30]

Early in February, the superintendents reported the center roof completed "except for painting and ornamental iron work," all floors laid, window frames all double-coated with paint and plumbing ready for placement of fixtures.[31]

In May, Browne wrote,

I take this opportunity to call your attention to the propriety of preparing [an] appartment [sic] in the Hospital for the reception of an insane or refractory patient. No provision for the same is made in the specifications. Communicating with the cellar, or unfinished portion of the basement is a small room, which size and position is well adapted for the purpose. This could be fitted with a wrought iron door and shutters, cast iron frames, bolts, locks and outside wooden door, etc., and the entire work rendered complete at a probable cost of three hundred and twenty five dollars ($325.00) in coin.[32]

Permission was granted for this, though Surgeon General William Maxwell Wood noted, "it is not considered necessary to have it provided with a wrought iron door or iron shutters."[33]

As can be imagined, there was much correspondence about specifics of construction—the need for mantles, changing water pipes from the specified concrete pipes to iron pipes, changes in the cistern; the details are numerous.

In March, the issue of a wash house and bakery arose. Browne sent a shopping list to the bureau, including washtubs, a furnace to heat flatirons, drying racks and an oven. Time was of the essence "as the building is advancing towards completion, should the Bureau authorize the above work, I would be pleased to receive notification by telegraph."[34] Approval arrived in early April.[35]

Three. A Firm Base for Health Care and the Doctors

By early April, the superintendents could state that most interior work was done and that "[the] bells and speaking tubes [no telephones yet!], and half of the lightening [sic] rods are fixed."[36]

The contract for extensive grading of the hospital grounds, a "add-in" project, was awarded to Charles Murphy of Vallejo for nearly half the estimated cost "owing to a competition between rival parties."[37]

On May 28, the superintendents wrote, "We have the honor to announce the completion of the Naval Hospital at this station."[38] They enclosed copies of the official report of acceptance by a board designated by the Commandant of the station. It was short and sweet:

> We have carefully examined the Naval Hospital just finished on this island, and have to report that the Contractors have fulfilled their contract in good faith and that the work throughout is exceedingly well done in all respects. All arrangements are complete and we think are admirable adapted for Hospital purposes with the latest improvements.

And this in the days before "grade inflation."

Completed but Not Finished

There were still myriad details to be attended to before the hospital would be ready to receive patients.

Commenting on the furniture in the old, temporary hospital—"the bedsteads are old, rickety and infested with insects," for example—Surgeon Browne opined that "the entire furniture is in a condition wholly unsuited for the use or economy of the new institution." Thereupon, he submitted his shopping list, "a complete outfit of articles."[39] The bureau approved 75 beds as being "a number sufficient for the present wants of the Station."[40] This number was revised downward yet again, as negotiations for furnishing the hospital advanced.[41]

A little later, responding to the bureau's request, he submitted his "list of employe's [sic] necessary to this Hospital in efficient operation"[42] and received approval for the following:[43]

Part I—The Early Years

1 Apothecary 1st Class	$1,000 [annual salary]
1 Chief Cook	$540
1 Asst	$480
3 Nurses @ $480[44]	$1,440
3 Washers @ $480	$1,440
2 Laborers @ $360	$720
1 Watchman	$360
2 Messroom Attendants @ $216	$432
1 Messenger	$144
1 Engineer	$1,000
1 Fireman	$500

The surgical operating table "from Mr. F.W. McIlroy of New York" was acknowledged "with pleasure" on August 19, as were the first volumes[45] for the library.[46]

At the end of August, Surgeon Browne submitted a detailed list of prospective hospital projects for the fiscal year ending June 30, 1872. Included were such items as trees for the hospital grounds ($1,700, including purchase, planting and "necessary support") and a surgeon's house, at a cost of $20,000.[47] As it turns out, the house would be a long time in coming. Hospital directors and their families set up housekeeping in one of the hospital wards during that long wait for proper quarters.

In October, Browne submitted a revised estimate for furnishing the hospital.[48] The nine-page document listed everything from medicine bottles to dishware to carpeting. His recapitulation: "For Dispensary—$196; for Bedding—$4413.75; for Furniture—$2985.50; for Crockery—$660.36; for Carpeting—$1152.25. Total—$9408.26 *in coin*" (emphasis mine. Legal tender paper money was still mistrusted in the gold country of California).

The logistics of the effort became complicated when the Surgeon General wrote Shipyard Commandant Goldsborough in late November. "Dispensary articles" were to be sent from the Naval Laboratory in New York City and articles of furniture from a Boston manufacturer. Surgeon General Wood went on,

Three. A Firm Base for Health Care and the Doctors

I will thank you to instruct Dr Browne to purchase [locally, in California—a third source of supply] only thirty (30) of each of the following named articles: iron bedsteads, hair mattresses, [illegible] mattresses, feather pillows and hair pillows. The Bureau has ordered from the manufacturer [a fourth supply source] several [15] fracture bedsteads, which will be sent out with the articles above referred to. Such of the excepted articles as are necessary to put the hospital partially in use to the extent of immediate requirements may be procured [in California].[49]

A couple of weeks later, Wood expressed his logistical frustration, writing again to Goldsborough:

I beg to say that there has been so much difficulty in obtaining specific information as to the articles required for the Naval Hospital, to avoid further delay it is thought necessary to put in operations only so much of the Hospital at Mare Island, as will meet the present demands.... If the thirty ward beds authorized are not sufficient for employes [sic] and patients, a sufficient number are to be obtained. The better class of furniture for officers' rooms, parlors, etc., will be sent from Boston, Mass. All things, with the exception of [a list of specified furniture and other items], and the dispensary articles and fracture beds, which are to be sent from the east, are to be procured in California.

A Horse and Wagon, and Coal for the Boiler

These few items needed to be supplied to ready the hospital for patients: a horse, wagon and harness (Browne: "Owing to the distance of the Hospital from the Navy Yard proper, it is necessary that provision be made for the transportation of supplies and the sick, independent of other departments, not only by reason of economy, but for accommodation and expediency"), approved "at a cost not to exceed the estimate [of $655]," on December 24[50]; 300 tons of "Pennsylvania (Scranton) coal"[51] at $13.50 per ton, approved on December 28.[52]

And at Long Last

In February 1871: "Letter No. 2" (I never found "Letter No. 1") from "U.S. Naval Hospital Mare Island, Cal.," dated February 1, 1871, put it succinctly, "Sir: I have the honor to report this Institution ready

Part I—The Early Years

> No. 2.
>
> U.S. Naval Hospital
> Mare Island, Cal.
> February 1st 1871.
>
> Sir:
>
> I have the honor to report this Institution ready for the reception of patients.
>
> I am, very respectfully
> Yr. obdt. servant
> Jno. M. Browne
> Surgeon in charge.
>
> Wm. M. Wood Esq. M.D.
> Chief of Bur. of Med & Surgery
> Washington, D.C.

Letter, Surgeon John Browne to Head of the Bureau of Medicine and Surgery, 1871. National Archives, Washington, D.C.

for the reception of patients. I am, very respectfully Yr obdt servant, John Browne, Surgeon in charge." The sailor who had his shattered hip removed in the temporary hospital walked out of this one a few weeks later.

Three. A Firm Base for Health Care and the Doctors

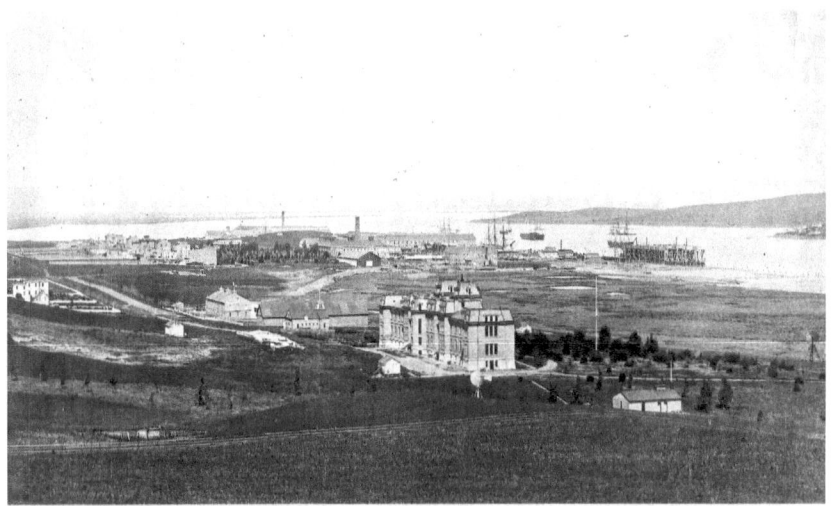

Panorama of Naval Hospital, Mare Island Naval Ship Yard, circa 1873. U.S. Navy Photo. National Archives, San Bruno, California.

Nearly 17 years after Commander Farragut established the Navy Yard at Mare Island, the hospital called for in his original planning document finally became a reality.

FOUR

A Hospital in Technological Transformation, 1871–1898

The *Vallejo Evening Chronicle* was brief and to the point in its description, on February 1, 1871, of the opening of the comparatively palatial new hospital on Mare Island: "NAVAL HOSPITAL—The new sick quarters at Mare Island were opened today, and arrangements have been made for the reception of *Saginaw*'s crew, should they require medical treatment on their arrival."[1]

The Navy Yard log describes a lovely February day: "Temperature at meridian [noon] 55, Weather Clear and Pleasant, Wind light from the S.W."[2] The facility received its inaugural patients in transfer from its predecessor, the "temporary hospital." The former granary was downgraded to a dispensary and medical stores facility.

On February 5, Surgeon John M. Browne—the first Medical Officer to serve on Mare Island—now the hospital director, could report 16 patients in hospital, with 14 vacant beds.[3] By the end of the month, the hospital census was 29 patients with just 1 empty bed.[4] The hospital was off to a busy start. It would remain busily full for the next two and a half decades. In this sense, some things about hospitals—the need to care for people—had not lessened. But over the next quarter century, the means for providing the care increased and changed substantially.

At the time of its opening, the hospital had some very "natural" limitations to its effectiveness. It depended on local rainfall for its water supply, with run-off from the roof routed to two cisterns near its foundation. The hospital relied on large windows (referred to as "lights" then) for daytime lighting; at night, lamps burning kerosene provided illumination. Heat came from the sun in the summer and from fireplaces and radiators heated by a coal-fired boiler during the cool Northern California winters. Patients called for assistance by crying out (if they were enlisted men in the wards) or shaking a handheld bell (the sick officers in their private rooms). Staff communicated through a system of bells and voice tubes. Messengers carried word by foot or by horse if a sailor at the waterfront or a Navy Yard worker was injured and required transport to the mile-distant hospital for care. Surgery, when required, was performed in a conference room temporarily converted for surgical use. If the need arose at night, patient and surgeon had to await the rising sun.

By the end of the century, all this had changed. Through a sweeping technological transformation, the quality of life and care were markedly different, and both surgeons and patients now had a glimpse of a world where men exerted substantial control over their environment.

Water, a Constant Worry

The precarious nature of the hospital water supply became apparent very early in the life of the new facility. Less than two months after opening, Browne wrote to the bureau to report that just 11 inches of rain had fallen during the wet season,[5] and the two cisterns contained only 16 inches of water, despite applying "the greatest practicable economy" in the use of that precious resource. He proposed installing a still—at a cost of $500 in coin—capable of producing 1,200 gallons of cool water per day, for which he did "respectfully solicit your favorable consideration of a method apparently well calculated to meet the urgency of the case."[6] A few days later, he submitted a bid by local contractor David Stoddart to install the still, a windmill for pumping salt water to the still, and a sunken 300 gallon tank for the system, for a total cost of $1,858. The bureau granted approval for the project in May and approved an additional payment

Part I—The Early Years

for circulating pumps in July.[7] Surgeon Browne signed the contract with Stoddart early in September, and he accepted the completed project, at a cost of $1,850, on October 13, 1871.

But another problem appeared in November. A windless period led to "the complete exhaustion of the water in our 'cisterns' from inability to use the 'condenser' during a calm of ten days, whereby our supply of 'salt water' was cut off." The new hospital director, Surgeon G.W. Woods, reported that he had purchased a high-capacity "fire pump," which he placed in service "for the purpose of using an abandoned 'Well,' in a ravine near the 'Hospital,' capable of furnishing 800 gals. of brackish water per day," as supply of water for the still.[8] A month later, Woods, describing problems with clogged drainpipes due largely to the lack of toilet flushing—a consequence of rigorous water conservation—proposed installation of a wind pump over the brackish well to provide water to permit the toilets to be regularly flushed, even in times requiring the most rigorous efforts of water conservation.[9] The bureau approved this expedience after duly receiving estimates for the work in February 1872.[10]

There things stood until Surgeon Browne, back in charge of the hospital after a tour as Surgeon of the Pacific Fleet, wrote in his August 1877 Estimate for Repairs and Improvements for Fiscal Year 1878,

> The supply of water caught from the roof is entirely inadequate for the requirement, necessitating the employment of salt-water, obtained from the Strait and pumped into the towers containing tanks, for baths, flushing of water closets, sewers, etc., thereby deteriorating all the water pipes throughout the building, and if persisted in will before long render necessary their replacement at a large expense. The Navy Yard is supplied by water from Vallejo, conducted in pipes to within 2800 feet of the Hospital, which distance, if traversed by two-inch pipe, would bring the Hospital, grounds & stable in possession of a sufficient supply of water. The estimated cost of pipe and labor is $700.[11]

Upon encountering silence from the bureau on the matter, Browne upped the ante in a letter to the bureau on December 7. With his reiteration of the dire water situation, he attached a letter from the captain of the yard, P.C. Johnson, who wrote, "As Captain of the

Four. A Hospital in Technological Transformation, 1871–1898

Yard, it is a part of my duty to take precautions against, and to provide means for extinguishing fire. The hospital is the only building that is deficient in respect to water. While the Yard is provided with three steam fire engines, they could not be of any use there as your cisterns are empty." He added, "Perhaps you may think it unnecessary for me to interest myself in regard to the hospital, as it is not under my charge, but if it takes fire, I strongly suspect that you would be glad to have assistance from the fire department of the yard, which would be unable to give you any with your cisterns empty." Johnson recommended using a "pipe connected with the main pipes of the yard for the purpose of keeping your cisterns full at all times" and added that although a two-inch pipe would be "sufficiently large for that purpose," one of four inches, "the size of the yard mains—would be much better." This recommendation received the commandant's endorsement, and he forwarded it to the bureau with his own respectful request that the bureau act on it because it was "of the utmost importance for the preservation of the Hospital and other property in case of fire."[12] The bureau resistance collapsed, and approval for the two-inch connector was sent west at the end of the month.[13]

Even a municipal source for water was no assurance of uninterrupted supply, and Hospital Director Somerset Robinson submitted requisitions to purchase water in July and again in December 1883. Faced with a critical shortage, he wrote early in December,

> I wish particularly to get the attention of the Bureau of Medicine and Surgery to the condition of this building in consequence of prolonged draught. We can no longer rely upon the Vallejo Water Co. to supply us as they exhausted their Lake in July 1883, and the people of that same village see how they would be exposed in case of flames. The use of the water from the Napa Creek has these objections, namely, expense in getting it to this building and subsequent harm to our cisterns and scaling of our pipes. The water which we purchase from the Spring Valley Water Company at the high rate of one and a half cents per gallon, and which will probably be higher on the next purchase, leaves considerable earthy sediment in our tower-tanks which are difficult to cleanse. Therefore, after three weeks of mature consideration and many consultations, I am of the belief that the surest, cheapest and best water is to be supplied us by process of distillation. To effect this

Part I—The Early Years

> most needful and immediate work it is required to get the loan of one No 5 Worthington pump, and one, at present, unfinished boiler from the Bureau of Steam Engineering, and in addition thereto the following articles by purchase, namely [lists items—including 2,500 feet of pipe—and labor to total $3,592.00]. The economy of getting our water supply from the Napa Creek, the distance of which from this building is indicated by the pipe asked, is that there will be no waste of water. The condenser need only be run in the rainless season. By purchase we may have water of a less desirable kind in our cisterns when the rains come.[14]

The commandant of the yard assisted during this crisis by permitting hospital personnel to run the power lighter[15] *Atlas* up the San Joaquin River to obtain fresh water. Robinson requested that the bureau pay for additional personnel for pumping the water from the lighter to the hospital cisterns, at a cost of $200—"payment in full for 60,000 to 70,000 gallons of water—and will supply the requisition much cheaper than by purchase in San Francisco."[16] The request for $200 received telegraphic approval from the bureau on December 18. The commandant of the yard followed up on the water situation by reporting in May 1884, "that by the strictest care and economy in the use of water at this Yard, the necessity for the purchase [of water] on requisition no 26, approved by the Bureau Dec 12 1883, has not arisen, and the requisition may be considered cancelled."[17]

Clearly, however, unless and until the problem of water supply in times of drought was solved, the water situation at the hospital would remain precarious. Even during years with normal waterfall, the summer months continued to be a time of water shortage within the hospital compound. Dr. Robinson was compelled to requisition water to refill the cisterns in September 1884 (with a 21-day supply remaining)[18] and communicated to the bureau a month later to request a water meter and gate (valve) be placed in the main water pipe for the yard—that ran right in front of the hospital—writing, "If this work be done, the Vallejo Water Co. will furnish the Hospital with water daily, at the same rate it now furnishes the Navy Yard—about 41 cents per 1000 gallons." He went on,

> We have depended so far this year upon the amount collected in our cisterns last winter and upon water furnished from time to time from that

Four. A Hospital in Technological Transformation, 1871–1898

collected in the large reservoir on the Navy Yard. These supplies are now exhausted and they have never been sufficient to allow of any irrigation whatever in the hospital ground. Many of the shrubs and plants are in great need of water. As it can be obtained at such a reasonable rate from the Vallejo Water Company, where the supply is abundant, I respectfully request that the Hospital be connected by means of the meter ... referred to.[19]

He promptly received permission from the bureau for the water meter and connection to the yard water distribution system.[20]

The meter and connection were duly installed, but still the situation was unsatisfactory because, it turned out, the two-inch line put in was simply too small. After testing the flow of water and proving that it took several hours for a flow of water to reach the hospital compound once the valve to the hospital line was opened, and after telegraphic inquiry from bureau to commandant about the advisability in installing the larger pipe (Belknap: "I recommend laying a new four-inch pipe as the best & only method of getting sufficient water supply"), and after convening a board of inspection ("You will examine the Water System of the Naval Hospital, and report ... the best and most economical manner of improving it so as to make the water service more satisfactory and reliable than it is at present, especially for such emergencies as now exist owing to the limited supply of water to be obtained from the contractor by reason of the light rainfall of the past two years"), the bureau approved, by telegram and letter, an extension, using four-inch pipe of the yard water system to the hospital cisterns in May 1888.[21] The work was completed on July 7, 1888.

A month later, Hospital Director Albert L. Gihon wrote to requisition a length of garden hose "to enable me to make use of the full amount of 166,666⅔ gallons of water per month, which I am instructed by the Commandant must be regularly delivered to the Hospital during the current fiscal year. I shall be very glad of this much needed opportunity of improving the lawns immediately surrounding the Hospital and the grounds within the Hospital Park, by irrigation."[22]

Medical Inspector Adrian Hudson wrote in November 1888,

Part I—The Early Years

indicating the need for an additional cistern to store water needed during the dry summer months. He went on to say that the 166,666 gallons per month were "not used in winter" and "not enough in summer." The bureau took the matter under consideration.[23] Hudson followed up with another missive in March 1889, reiterating the need for additional water storage and expressing concern about the reliability of the city water supply which, because of low winter rainfall, could be cut off from the hospital.

In August, John Mills Browne, once the medical director in charge of the Mare Island Hospital and now the Surgeon General of the Navy, took the matter to the Secretary of the Navy:

> Medical Director Hudson, in charge of the Naval Hospital at Mare Island, Cal, recommends the construction of a cistern for the storage of the excess of water received from the opposite town of Vallejo, not only for protection from fire, but whenever by the presence of drought, which was feared last summer, the Water Company could not give the usual supply.
>
> The cistern proposed is required to be sixty-five feet in diameter by ten feet in depth. Parties in San Francisco estimate the cost at $3,500.00 *or with a concrete roof $4,500.00* The Department of Yards and Docks at Mare Island estimates the cost at $7,917.15.[24]

The precarious water supply was again taken up in the Surgeon General's annual report to the Secretary of the Navy in October 1889:

> A cistern for the stowage of water to contain 200,000 gallons, is needed, placed upon declivity in rear of hospital, to enable the delivery of water into the two principal stories of the hospital without the labor and cost of pumping from present reservoir into lower tanks as must now be done. Serious difficulties would follow any accident to the main of the Vallejo Water Co. which crosses the Napa Straits, by preventing the delivery of water; or the sudden use of a large amount in case of fire, or, in event of a water famine (which was threatened this season) would demand a reserve of water in storage. A permanent advantage would be the saving of water supplied in winter from Vallejo, under existing arrangements, in excess of needs. An additional cistern would prevent the use of one of those already built for containing the supply of drinking water caught from the roof, thereby having a pure water in place of the impure water received from Vallejo.[25]

The assurance of a reliable water supply first appears in a report from Hospital Director G.W. Woods. Responding to a circular letter

Four. A Hospital in Technological Transformation, 1871–1898

from the bureau requesting a statement of details about all the naval hospitals, he comments about the water supply:

> Two pumps serve for raising water from the cisterns to tanks in each mansard tower, whence it is distributed by an elaborate system of pipes to all buildings, and throughout the grounds. The two cisterns have a united capacity of 121,527.96 gallons, and that of the tanks is 5600 gallons. The water is brought from an artificial pond, in the suburbs of Vallejo, through a sub-marine pipe, and it's [sic] potability is often questionable; but a supply of pure water will be introduced from Green Valley Falls during the year 1894.[26,27]

Woods, sending input for the Secretary of the Navy's annual report to Congress for fiscal year 1894, reported, "An important sanitary feature has been the introduction, during the past year, of 'Green Valley Water' for supplying the Navy Yard and Hospital. The supply is practically unlimited, and with a pressure sufficiently great to reach far above the highest buildings."[28]

At this, the problem of insufficient or unreliable water for the hospital appears to have vanished: no further correspondence on the topic appears in the records of the bureau until around World War II.

From Kerosene Lamps to Gas to Electricity

Although Surgeon Browne anticipated that gas lighting would be introduced to the new hospital soon after its completion,[29] the hospital was lighted only by lamps burning kerosene oil. In fact, Hospital Director Woods, responding to a bureau inquiry eight months after the hospital opened its doors for business, noted that these lamps, in three wards, burned an average of 35 gallons per month, at a cost of $25.[30] Woods was answering an inquiry from Washington in which the bureau informed him that the installation of a "Butler's Gas Works" for the manufacture of illuminating gas for the hospital compound was under consideration.[31]

In April 1872, more than a year after the hospital started up, Surgeon General Jonathan M. Foltz wrote hospital Officer in Charge J.S. Dungan directing him to "confer with the agent of the 'Butler Gas Works' now at Mare Island" and, after deciding the needs of

Part I—The Early Years

the apparatus, to solicit bids for construction of a building "to be of brick"[32] to house it. The lowest of four bidders—at $3,878—was Charles Murphy of Vallejo, and on July 5, 1872, Dungan reported completion of the project. "The Gas House," he wrote, "is a substantial building with a solid foundation. A site for the House was selected in the ravine at the south end of the Hospital, and distant 154 feet from it." Dungan went on to request purchase of the pipe necessary to connect the gasworks with the hospital and stable and to purchase the gas fixtures for the hospital: 52 chandeliers, 4 wall lights, 15 pendants, 77 brackets, 7 droplights and 2 lampposts.[33] He later added "two lights, with globes, to be placed over the front door, main entrance, of the Hospital" to his wish list. Responding to a request "for an estimate of the cost of the articles, in detail," Dungan submitted the list, with prices "in gold coin." He commented,

> "I can buy them in San Francisco at an advance in New York prices of only the premium on gold."[34] He went on "The premium about equals the freight between New York and San Francisco, but thus avoid [sic] the risk of breakage and other damages. Two houses in S.F. [writer's abbreviation] have very large stocks in hand to select from.... I would like to make this selection—in which I take much interest—to adapt them to the Hospital, the rooms, halls, wards &c."[35]

Of interest is the request of "2 4-light Pendants" for the operating room on the third floor. He received bureau approval for purchase in San Francisco early in September.

By the end of September, Dungan reported that "Mr. H.N. Ames, the Agent for Hutchinson Brothers, of Baltimore Maryland" had completed construction of the Butler gas generator. The "apparatus," he wrote, "consists of a bench of four generators, and a holder of 3400 [cubic] feet." Dungan further added that the Navy Yard gasworks superintendent had declared the generator "to be well constructed, and in excellent condition." Soon thereafter, Dungan acknowledged the bureau's approval to appoint a fireman for the gasworks at $750 per year. By the end of November, the gashouse had been duly connected by pipe to the hospital. It took until May 1873 for all the gas fixtures in the hospital and stables to be fully installed. Fixtures were placed in all public spaces, workspaces, wards, quarters, on the

Four. A Hospital in Technological Transformation, 1871–1898

hospital grounds, the gashouse itself, the stable and at the hospital main entrance.

The gas lighting appears to have worked efficiently and durably, for there is no correspondence concerning illumination of the hospital until May 1881, when Medical Director George Peck (in charge of the hospital), in forwarding a proposal to connect the hospital to the Vallejo (municipal) Gas Light Company, wrote, "A careful consideration of the subject leads me to believe that a saving to the Government of 59 per cent, as compared with the cost of our present manufacture, can be made through the introduction of Vallejo gas."[36] Surgeon General Philip Skinner Wales prudently requested more information—the quantity of gas used, the cost of manufacture and the quality of illumination produced by the product of the Vallejo Gas Light Company compared with that of local manufacture—and he requested Peck's recommended course of action.

On May 26, Peck provided the requested information: "During the year ending March 31, 1881, there were 99725 cubic feet of gas consumed of 22 candlepower, manufactured at a cost of $1124.39, exclusive of labor. This amount includes oil, fuel, wear and tear of apparatus, etc., and gives an average cost of $11.27 per 1000 cubic feet."

He went on,

> The Vallejo Gas Light Co's gas is of 17 candle power, and is offered to us for $3.00 per 1000 cubic feet. If it were 22 candlepower as is the gas we make, it would be worth $3.89 per 1000 cubic feet—at this price there would be a saving of $7.38 per 1000 cubic feet, as compared with the cost of ours. The lighting of the Hospital at present is unsatisfactory, because of the use of three-felt[37] burners, necessitated by the quality and character of our gas and the excessive cost of manufacture. The best burners (five-felt) with Vallejo gas, will secure us a steadier, and more brilliant illumination. The appearance and comfort of the house would be improved by a better lighting, which, it must be remembered, would entail a greater consumption of gas if the Vallejo Co's product were used: but with this increased consumption the cost would yet fall below that made by us, and I think we may count on a saving of at least 40 to 50 per cent.
>
> I advise, in view of the above facts, the discontinuance of the present method of supply, and recommend the use of Vallejo Co's gas, as economical and conducive to well being of the patients and inmates of the hospital.[38]

Part I—The Early Years

There the matter lay until September, when Peck once again brought up the idea of using municipal gas. This time, he enclosed a letter from the Vallejo Gas Light Company offering to lay hospital-provided gas pipe at no cost to the government.[39] Annual estimates for repairs dated October 1, 1881, listed "gas, pipe, for connecting with main of Vallejo Gaslight Co.—$990."[40]

Faced with the bureau's silence on the matter, Peck again wrote on the matter in June 1882. He submitted a proposal from the Vallejo Gas Light Company to supply and lay pipe for $1,250 and from the Central Gas Company of San Francisco to construct a new apparatus "of the Hanlon pattern, for generating gas from petroleum."[41] In August, he wrote to say the gas retorts and gas holder were in decrepit condition and "liable to give way at any time."[42] The bureau responded indicating that "the condition of the appropriations prevents the Bureau from authorizing the arrangement proposed" and went on with a request for the "names of two or more parties to whom it can write for proposals for repairing the gas holders and retorts."[43]

Peck sent names of three parties from Vallejo and a fourth from San Francisco. On September 23, he again wrote to Surgeon General Wales:

> I have already expressed to the Bureau the need for immediate action in this matter so urgently that I am at a loss to know how to represent it better.... In the present condition of our apparatus the amount of oil expended to produce a given quantity of gas is more than double that required by the same apparatus when new; and probably apparatus of more recent design than Butler's would be more economical still. Thus, it is estimated that the apparatus of the Central Gas co. of San Francisco, whose proposal was submitted to the Bureau some time ago, is more advantageous than the system we now use. The repairs to our apparatus would be, from what I can learn, so costly as to be of doubtful economy except as related to the gas-holder....
> If [the Vallejo Gas Light Company] proposal is accepted we could light the Hospital without regard to the gas-holder, only retaining it as a reservoir to use in case of accident to the supply pipe which runs under the water of Vallejo strait [really, the Napa River, which separates the city of Vallejo from the island].[44]

To emphasize the urgency of his problem, Medical Director Peck telegraphed the bureau on September 21: *Gas furnace broken*

Four. A Hospital in Technological Transformation, 1871–1898

down. Requisition forwarded fire brick to repair. Approval requested by Telegraph.[45]

Two days later, the Surgeon General laconically replied in a letter, "The bureau has this day written for proposals for repairing the gas holder and retorts at the Naval Hospital, Mare Island, Cal., and when they are received it will decide whether the repairs shall be made or the offer of the Vallejo Gas Light Company be accepted."[46]

The Vallejo company weighed in on the matter when, in October, president of Vallejo Gas Light Company E.J. Wilson[47] wrote the Surgeon General,

> In view of the precarious condition of the machine for manufacturing Gas at the Naval Hospital at Mare Island, and the further fact that the Bureau of Medicine and surgery [sic] is lacking in funds, the Vallejo Gas Light Company will lay down the pipe to connect the Hospital with their Gas main on the Navy Yard and will furnish Gas such as is now supplied to the navy yard [sic] under their Contract at three ($3.00) dollars per thousand [cubic] feet. This pipe will be laid in land belonging to the Government, and in due time we propose to ask Congress to appropriate money to re-emburse [sic] us for our expense in laying down the pipe.[48]

The bureau did not reply.

Silence also resulted from Peck's requisition in December for labor to construct eight gas retorts at "probable cost, sixty ($60.00) dollars."[49]

Eight months later, Peck once again took up the gas supply matter:

> During the past month, the Vallejo Gas Light Company have laid a main to the marine Barrack, within a comparatively short distance of this Hospital. In response to a letter from me, the company have offered to connect the Hospital with this main, for $370, and to furnish gas thereafter for $3.00 per thousand cubic feet. During the past fiscal year to manufacture the gas used, we have paid $1216.47 for oil alone, to say nothing of repairs, or the cost of making [the gas]. At the prices noted, $370.00 for connecting, and $450 for years supply of gas (150,000 [cubic] ft at $3.00 per 000.) the saving will be apparent. The light we can thus obtain will be much more desirable on account of cleanliness and safety, and we shall gain in economy of labor and additional room for our laundry.[50]

The bureau, hanging tough, replied that it "adhears [sic] to its original proposition; that if the Gas company will lay the Main, the

53

Part I—The Early Years

bureau will agree to take the gas at the rate of $3.00 per m. feet."[51] The gas company replied that at $3.00 per 1,000 cubic feet, the profits would be "too small to justify so large an outlay and in this particular case it would take years for the profits to cover the original cost of the mains." The company went on to detail that the mains to the Navy Yard and to the Marine barracks nearby the hospital had been laid at government expense and that they would be "willing to negotiate with the Hospital upon the same terms as we have with the other branches of the service."[52]

In November, apparently resigned to the fact that the hospital would continue to produce its own gas but still in desperate need of upgraded, gas-generating equipment, Robinson wrote the bureau to indicate that the Department of Steam Engineering on the Navy Yard had patterns for casting new retorts; he requested permission to have that department cast them, at a cost of $50 for the labor.[53] Shortly thereafter, the bureau notified the yard commandant that new retorts for the hospital gas generator had been ordered for shipment to the Navy Yard.[54]

But Navy Yard officials persisted in their efforts to get municipal gas delivered to the hospital. Early in February 1884, Yard Commandant John Henry Russell telegraphed the bureau to indicate that he was extending the yard's gas service to the stables, nearby the hospital, and that "Medical Inspector Robinson requests authority to extend to hospital three hundred and fifty feet." He added, "Recommend telegraph answer."[55]

Apparently, the Secretary of the Navy got into the act because, in a February 14 letter to the bureau, Commandant Russell, citing the "Hon. Secretary of the Navy authorizing" the extension of gas service to the hospital, detailed the need for one-and-a-half-inch pipe to be laid at "an estimated cost of $450—labor and material." He added, "As the statements of expense of the present system of supply are in the Bureau's files and showing it to be greatly excessive, I earnestly recommend the expenditure now proposed."[56] The bureau relented on February 21, authorizing the work at a cost "not to exceed $450."[57]

The laying of pipe and connections moved quickly along, and

Four. A Hospital in Technological Transformation, 1871–1898

Medical Director Robinson submitted his first bill from the Vallejo Gas Light Company "for gas consumed during the second quarter ending June 30, 1884" on July 4.

And there things lay, except for routine affairs of gas pipe, gas lamp and gas meter maintenance, until 1889, when on March 19, Hudson wrote to the bureau:

> I am informed that an appropriation for supplying electric light to the Mare Island Navy Yard has been made available. I beg to suggest, therefore that the Bureau will consider the propriety of connecting the Hospital grounds with the system of lighting the Yard and if it be regarded as desirable to make such arrangements as may be necessary with the Bureau of Yards and Docks where I understand the plans are being prepared.

Surgeon General William K. Van Reypen promptly replied in the affirmative:

> The Bureau has communicated with the Chief of the Bureau of Yards and Docks, and is informed that when the electric light plant is established in the Mare Island Yard provision will be made for furnishing sufficient current to light the Hospital. Will you be pleased to inform the Bureau as to the number of lights of 16 candle power that will be required to take the place of the gas lights now in use in the Hospital, including outbuildings and grounds under charge of the Bureau of Medicine and Surgery [sic].

Hudson noted in reply that the hospital used 280 gas burners, but given the increased efficiency of incandescent lights, the number of fittings could be "diminished in rooms at present supplied by chandiliers [sic] and gas burners by about fifty."[58] In his October 7, 1891, annual report to the Secretary of the Navy, the Surgeon General commented,

> An electric light plant has been installed at the Navy Yard, and an extension of this system to the hospital will require no additional boiler and dynamo power; only independent wires, transformers, switch boards, etc., will be needed. As it is expected that gas will be used except at the Marine Barracks and hospital, it is apprehended the service may not be satisfactory, hence the desirability of lighting with electricity, which the Bureau hopes to accomplish.[59]

In July 1892, the bureau received the hospital director's "wish list" for fiscal year 1893. Number one on that list was "the introduction of 'Electric Light.'" In his accompanying memorandum, Woods wrote,

Part I—The Early Years

> I place the electric light as first in importance for these reasons, viz., that the hospital is the only customer, at present, of the "Vallejo Gas Company" on the "Yard," the gas being received through a sub-marine pipe, and a pump, engine, and tender is maintained at the end of the Georgia Street wharf [which lay across the Napa River from the island], for its delivery. At any time, the Company may discontinue this service as being unprofitable, or increase the price, and should the sub-marine pipe be rendered unserviceable by breakage—a not uncommon accident—or otherwise, it would cease, as the pipe will certainly not be repairable at the expense of the Company.

He added, "I am officially informed that the electric plant of the 'Yard' is of sufficient power to supply the incandescent lamps required in all the buildings under our control, and three arc-lamps [for illumination of hospital ground]."[60] Woods also supplied the bureau with some proposed details: The hospital would need 235 incandescent lamps, the laundry 10. Five lights would serve the stable, and the newly built director's house would require 75. The cost of electricity for each of these "16 candle-power lights"[61] would be one cent per hour.[62]

From here, things moved with extraordinary dispatch, with bids for "wiring and poles for power to be delivered from Yard electric plant, internal wiring and fixtures, switches and cut-outs to protect the wiring [fusing], 235 in hospital proper, 10 in laundry, 5 in stable. $3425. //signed// Geo E Hanscom." On December 19, Woods wrote the bureau to report that the electrical work would be completed by Christmas Eve and that the electrical hookup to the yard electrical plant would occur "but a few days later." He inquired of the bureau if, once he had electricity, the gas service should be discontinued.

The bureau demurred briefly but on January 13, 1893, wired Woods their permission to "begin use of electric lights whenever plant is entirely ready." Woods replied that the connection with the yard system had been completed on the 10th.[63]

Thus, in almost exactly 22 years, doctors, staff and patients experienced candles and daylight, to gas, to electrical lighting. One can only surmise what changes this evolution of technology made in their lives.

Four. A Hospital in Technological Transformation, 1871–1898

From Speaking Tubes, Bells and Runners to Telephone Communications

In his April 1870 construction report, Surgeon Browne, the construction supervisor, noted that the "bells and speaking tubes" had been installed. Speaking tubes were commonplace in naval vessels, office buildings and even private homes. One merely yelled into the funnel-shaped mouthpiece at one end; the sound was conducted by a (typically) two-inch pipe to a funnel on the other end, where the recipient, perhaps several rooms or floors away, could hear and respond. A system of bells often accompanied the tubes—a way of getting the attention of the person at the other end.[64]

Enlisted men, when hospitalized, occupied beds in the hospital wards. These men probably benefited from the more or less constant presence of a hospital attendant nearby, who could respond to their verbal calls for assistance. For hospitalized officers, the situation was different, as described by Surgeon Browne in an early 1879 letter to the bureau:

> The rooms set aside for the use of invalid Officers are comparatively remote from the necessary stations of the regular Nurses and Watchmen, & even if they were not, the fact that it is impracticable for an officer to keep his door constantly open renders it impossible to hear, even at a short distance, the hand-bells habitually used in our Hospitals. Quite recently we have had four Officers under treatment, one of whom was confined to his bed & it was necessary in the case of this last named patient, to detail men solely to remain near his door, day & night, in order to hear his bell. To perform such duty as this we must either call upon patients, who through indifference or lack of intelligence cannot always be relied upon, or employ a special attendant.[65]

Among the hospital list of civil employees in 1872 was "1 Messenger."[66] The hospital lay about a mile from the Navy Yard. Any communication to the yard or to the ships, including the receiving ship USRS *Independence*, required a runner or messenger to walk or run that mile. Similarly, if a worker were injured on the Navy Yard or a sailor on the waterfront taken seriously ill, a runner would have to be dispatched that distance to the hospital to summon aid.

Part I—The Early Years

Communication with the wider world was no simpler. Of course, one had the post office. Letters typically took a week or more to traverse the expanses of the continent. Telegraph was quicker (overnight service was typical), but it was inconvenient—the telegraph office was located on Sacramento Street in downtown Vallejo. One had to hike the mile from the hospital to the waterfront, take a boat across the Napa River that lay between the island and the city, then hike nearly another mile to the telegraph office. And telegraphy was expensive: at about a dollar for a ten-word telegram.[67] All of these were good reasons for the surgeons at the hospital to request electrical communications as they became available.

The first step was to install a system of "electric bells and annunciators" that officer patients could use to summon assistance. Using the argument of economy (the cost of purpose-hired special attendants would pay for the system in about three months), Browne, now officer in charge of the hospital for the third time, requested approval to purchase the device from New York and batteries to run it in San Francisco.[68]

The arrangements for the enlisted patients remained the same.

The first request for telephones came in a letter written by Browne in June 1879. At no expense, Browne had placed poles and two lines, one of which was connected to the Gate House and General Office at the Navy Yard. However, until he had receivers and transmitters, the lines were of no use. He emphasized that the telephone would permit the service of the steam fire engine "immediately," and "by means of this communication the presence of invalids or supplies at the Gate House, waiting for transportation will be known, and thus obviate unnecessary trips of the wagon or ambulance." Rental of two receivers and two transmitters at a cost of $40 per year was promptly approved by the bureau.[69] In 1880, renewal of the rental, from the Pacific Bell Telephone Company, was approved. By 1887, Hospital Director Gihon indicated that phone connections outside the island were available, reporting a phone call from the superintendent of the Vallejo City Water Company.[70] I did not find correspondence in the file to confirm the use of the telephone for "long distance"—for example, to Washington, D.C.—communications at this time.

The Occasional Operating Room Transformed to Purpose-Built Space for Surgery

It appears that one modernization that the naval hospital medical staff did not actively solicit was a purpose-built operating room. From the hospital's opening, surgical operations were performed in the first-floor conference room which was converted to a surgery on an as-needed basis. Woods described the setup in a letter to Surgeon General Newton L. Bates in March 1896:

> The room ... is a double room ... on the first floor, easily accessible from the two lower wards, and adjacent to the elevator.... It is completely lighted from the South-West, throughout the entire day, and needs no illumination from above. The room ... is now in use as an Operating and Board room. Its dimensions are: length, 21 feet; width, 14 feet; height, 14 feet, 6 inches. The windows are two in number, each 8 ft. 10 in × 3 ft. 6 in. in dimensions and terminate 2 ft. 10 in. from the floor. It is already provided with hot, and cold water, a porcelain sink, and a stand for aseptic solutions, furnished with proper bottles, and is heated by steam. The floor is linoleum, and the walls are hard-finished.[71]

The bureau, in the meanwhile, based on experience at the Philadelphia naval hospital, had decided that all operating rooms in naval hospitals should meet a standard of construction and equipment. The Surgeon General wrote to the Mare Island commandant, "To meet the requirements of modern aseptic surgery, I will thank you to direct the Medical Officer in charge of the Naval Hospital under your command[72] to have the room set aside for operating purposes ... prepared." He then went on to provide very specific guidance including paint brand (Rinald's) and colors, and furnishings. The Surgeon General also called for the installation of "a sufficient number of electric lights ... properly located to insure ample artificial light during an operation, with a moveable burner [a throwback term to the recent days of gas lighting?] that can be used when required to reflect light into [body] cavities, or in using a laryngoscope or endoscope."[73]

Part I—The Early Years

Ventilation and heating of the room was to be left to the judgment of the Medical Officer in charge. Finally, the bureau went on to specify the equipment of the room, including a water sterilizer "to supply absolutely sterile water," and dressing and instrument sterilizers.

Despite some difficulty in obtaining the precise equipment specified, and using the operating room at the Waldeck Hospital in San Francisco as a guide, Hospital Director Woods gradually put the pieces together. In a letter to the Surgeon General on February 4, 1897 (not quite a year later), Woods reported, "The 'Operating Room' is now completely furnished, and in working order, having been used for an operation at night, on the 3rd inst. [the day before this letter], with great satisfaction."[74] One can only image the "great satisfaction" to both surgeon and patient that surgery now didn't have to wait until the sun's rays came pouring through the operating room windows to proceed with the operation.

In just one year, Naval Hospital, Mare Island, California, had made a giant step into the world of modern medicine and surgery: a purpose-built—and maintained—operating room.

Of significant note is that the hospital had received equipment but not the furniture for a bacteriology lab in conjunction with the operating room, as directed by the bureau. This latter facility was finally "institutionalized" by the bureau about 30 years after Joseph Lister's work proved the role of bacteria in causing surgical infection.

The Problem with 19th-Century Plumbing

Despite glowing reports of efficient and competent construction offered to the contractor—"the work throughout is exceedingly well done in all respects"[75]—problems with the plumbing, especially the toilets and sewer plumbing, soon became apparent. Less than a year after opening, Hospital Director G.W. Woods was prompted to complain about problems with clogged sewer lines due to small size, extreme water conservation which prevented flushing and, regarding the kitchen drains, their long and circuitous route. He requested approval to reroute the kitchen drains and to purchase a wind pump,

Four. A Hospital in Technological Transformation, 1871–1898

for $300 gold coin, "to assure enough water supply to permit regular flushing of the pipes."[76]

This pump was to be placed over a well located in the ravine immediately to the south of the hospital. In July 1872, Hospital Commander J.S. Dungan expanded the theme:

> I have been compelled to incur considerable expense to remove serious obstructions in the two main sewers, and in six drain pipes, in this Hospital. One of these sewers, composed of asphaltum cement, was melted by the steam and hot water from the boilers in the Engine Room. The circuitous course and a want of a proper descent, were, and still are, the causes of obstruction in the other sewer. These sewers are of insufficient size. Pipes from the Water Closets lead into them. The six leaden pipes from the sinks, bath room and water closet, were found defective in size, quality, angular turns and horizontal leads.

Rather than request permission to correct these problems, he asked for "forgiveness," having on his own initiative replaced these "by other pipes of superior quality and without the formers' defects." He added, "The immediate removal of the obstructions mentioned, and the repair of damages, were matters of imperative necessity."[77]

Apparently, Dungan anticipated more difficulties with the plumbing because in his proposed budget for fiscal year 1873–4, he entered a line item of $8,000, a princely sum, for "sewers and other drain pipes."

One wonders if these repairs were ever approved because in August 1875, Medical Inspector James Suddards was moved to provide in distasteful detail:

> I enclose herewith Estimates by E.G. Armstrong, Foreman & Machinist of the Department of Yards and Docks at this Yard, for repairs to Bath-tubs, Wash-Basins & Water Closets of this Hospital. These repairs have long been needed. The sinks in the Dispensary and other places were put in order by Med¹ Inspector Dungan. The condition of the water-closets &c enumerated above is such that further delay is scarcely possible. The "Bath-tubs," seven in number, were originally lined with Zinc, which has corroded to such an extent that it can no longer be repaired. Only one in the building can now be used at all, without danger of flooding all the immediate neighborhood. It is proposed to re-line them with sheet-lead, which will last for an indefinite period, and can be mended, if leaky, at a moment's notice. The "Water-Closets" were put in by the Contractor without being properly

Part I—The Early Years

trapped. The consequence is, that when the wind blows from certain quarters, such an offensive odor escapes as almost to drive everyone out of the building, and some of the wards are absolutely untenantable.

The same Contractor, I am credibly informed, furnished similar work to the City & County Hospital at San Francisco, and the authorities were put to the expense of from six to seven thousand dollars to remedy the Evil, just as we propose to do.

The pipes, "Tin & Lead," are for the purpose of carrying off the water &c from the Wash Basins, Urinals and Bath-tubs. As constructed, the pipes are too small, so that they are easily choked up, and the water does not run off. The Soil-pipe, heretofore of lead, has been nearly destroyed by rats. It is intended to replace it by one of iron. All the pipes moreover, will have a more perpendicular direction, so that all refuse matters, water or other, will have free egress to the main sewer.

His peroration was, "I deem the repairs mentioned of the most imminent necessity, and strongly recommend that I may be authorized to have them carried out."[78] The estimated cost would be $850 and take about a month to complete.

Browne wrote in his repairs want list in May 1879, "The necessity for ventilating the water-closets is urgent. The presence of sewer gas in one or more parts of the building is of almost daily occurrence." To this end, he proposed, "Ventilation of sewers & water-closets, by traps, & by pipes leading to the roof, at an estimated cost of $98."[79]

In October 1880, Navy Yard Commandant E.R. Colhoun joined the fray, writing to his civil engineer (with a copy to the bureau, of course),

> That the apparent need of additional ventilation, arose more from the imperfect apparatus of the Water-Closets and bad drainage than from defects in the building itself. The present plans of these water-closets are without water seals, except perhaps where the contrivances may exist in the discharge pipes, which is doubtful, thus serving but a very imperfect purpose, as experience here unmistakably demonstrates.

He recommended that the faulty pan water closets be replaced "with others of a more recent date and effective construction" and called for devices of the "Milne & Gants pattern."[80] The innovation of this toilet was a feature that permitted the bowl to be continually filled with water, thus preventing the backflow of sewer gas into the hospital.

Four. A Hospital in Technological Transformation, 1871–1898

The commandant went on to point out that the original sewer pipes, made from brick, were inclined to back up due to their general layout and settlement in their course. He recommended the old sewer piping be replaced with smooth vitrified ("stone ware") pipes, properly trenched and graded.[81]

The bureau entertained bids for the required plumbing work both from two Vallejo contractors and from Bartlett, Hayward and Co. (who were in the process of making improvements to the hospital heating and ventilating system) in July and August. Even at that, Medical Director Peck was prompted to write on September 1,

> On raising the floor of the basement of the hospital, preparatory to laying the pipes of the heating apparatus, etc., a breakage was found in the drain pipe, whereby the soil had become saturated for forty feet under the central portion of the building. Further examination showed that the sewer pipes outside the house are above the level of the drain-pipes leading into them, thus causing stagnation of sewage in them for a distance of twenty or thirty feet. The sewer which received the drainage of the house is of asphaltum, without sufficient inclination, and broken in places, discharging more or less into the adjacent soil, and causing part of the fecal odor which has been perceptible ever since I took charge of the Hospital. As far as can be judged the asphalt sewer is in a very frail condition: it crumbles readily under the hand, rats gnaw into it, etc.[82]

A pond of sewage under the cellar floor! I am taken with Peck's dispassionate description of the "fecal odor" that perfused the hospital. Peck's October 1, 1881, budget for the next fiscal year included a plumber's estimates for water closets, bathrooms, and so forth totaling $1,795.00.[83]

As if to punctuate the urgency of the sewer problem, Peck telegraphed the bureau on October 30, "FLOORS LIFTED IN LOWEST HALL TO CONNECT THE NEW SEWER EXPOSE FILTH FROM BROKEN CLOSETS AND WORN OUT SOIL PIPE. PLUMBING REPAIRS IMPERATIVELY NEEDED. ESTIMATED COST THREE HUNDRED DOLLARS. AUTHORITY TO EMPLOY LOWEST BIDDER REQUESTED BY TELEGRAPH."[84] With relief at receiving the bureau's approval, he wrote to expand the description: not only had asphaltum[85] sewer pipes disintegrated, but the old iron hopper toilets had rusted through, permitting sewage to fall directly to the

Part I—The Early Years

earth beneath the hospital. By early December, Peck could report to the Surgeon General,

> All the sewage and waste water of the house is now discharged by the shortest route into a single continuous cylindrical pipe, ten (10) inches in diameter, with the exception of the waste-water from the kitchen which escapes through a separate eight (8) inch pipe, in front of the house, as shown in the plan. The good effect of the new sewer is noticeable in the absence of foul odors, formerly constant, in the halls. The old sewer of asphaltum was simply an elongated cess-pool, having so little fall as to be choked and in many places, broken and crumbling. The drain and soil pipes were connected with the main by smaller asphaltum pipes beneath the basement floor. The drain pipes are now of lead and iron, and all joints with the sewer are outside the building, except the soil pipes, the joints of which are exposed to view at will by lifting a trap-door.

He put in another pitch to replace old toilets on the upper floors with "those having sufficient water-seal, with ducts connecting them to the Emerson ventilators in the roof, thus ensuring the removal of all offensive odors."[86]

Yet a year later, Peck was again moved to complain about the faulty water closets in the upper floors:

> I desire to call attention first of all to the necessity of new and improved water-closets throughout the house, except where a few have recently been put in. In the case of all except these last it is impossible to prevent offensive odors escaping and contaminating the air of the halls, wards, and private apartments. In some places the connections between soil-pipe and water closet have been loosened, and the pipe itself is so frail and corroded from long use that it is impossible to attempt repair.[87]

He submitted a request for $1,500 to effect the repairs in his fiscal year 1883–4 budget. And in January 1883, "herewith enclosed I transmit to the Bureau requisition in triplicate for six water-closets—Milne & Gant's patent—and labor and material for setting the same. The closets which the above are needed to replace are so worn and deteriorated by long use as to be no longer tolerable—they leak and are constantly offensive."[88]

Finally, the faulty toilets were replaced in fiscal year 1885–86. In 1887, the Milne & Gants toilets were found to be worn out and wasting water. That San Francisco firm now being out of business, Gihon

Four. A Hospital in Technological Transformation, 1871–1898

received permission to establish a board of survey to evaluate the toilets for replacement rather than repair. This board duly met and learned that elsewhere on the yard (for instance, in the officers' quarters), these water closets served quite well. The board laid much of the blame for the hospital's problems on incompetent maintenance by the hospital engineer. The board declined to recommend replacing the toilets.[89,90]

In February 1892, Bates wrote the bureau,

> In replacing the bath tubs in wards 1, 2 and 3 by new ones recently purchased, I found that the tubs made direct connections with waste pipes which were neither trapped nor ventilated. The bath room plumbing at each end of the building should be entirely renewed. This will involve 2" cast iron pipe with caulked joints from sewer to opening above roof, ventilated traps under each tub and the setting for four tubs.
>
> I inclose [sic] proposal from Mr John Brownlie of Vallejo to do the work for one hundred dollars. This offer is reasonable and I recommend that it be accepted, and the work ordered. A second proposal in duplicate is made by Mr Thomas Creighton, a plumber of Vallejo, is also inclosed [sic].[91] [I saw "noted" in red ink on the face of the letter "Req approved"]

The bureau saw the sad state of 19th-century plumbing through to complete remedy, though, in 1893, Surgeon General Browne wrote to the commandant of the yard on April 4,

> With the view of improving the sanitary condition of the Hospital under your command, the Bureau would be pleased to have you direct Medical Inspector G.W. Woods to report, at once, upon the condition of all water closets in the building, whether necessary to repair them, or whether, in the interest of health and economy, it might not be more expedient to have them replaced by new ones. If the latter is deemed necessary, you will direct Medical Inspector Woods to procure proposals from two or three reliable firms, the proposals to accompany requisition for repairs.[92]

One wonders if the Surgeon General remembers the sewer gas pervading the hospital when he had command of the place 17 years earlier! In any case, Woods promptly reported back that 11 closets of the "plug" (i.e., Milne & Gants) design were unsanitary, in part because they lacked a trap between bowl and sewer, so that when the plug was raised to permit emptying, sewer gas could escape into the room. He recommended that all 11 be replaced with "washout" toilets, properly fitted with traps underneath.[93]

Part I—The Early Years

Woods, in his statement of improvements for the fiscal year ending June 30, 1893, mentioned "nine siphon closets" had been installed at a cost of $400. Finally, the hospital was fitted out with 13 toilets of modern design, after 22 years in operation. End of story and end of correspondence on the matter.

The Facility and Staff Grow to Meet the Increasing Needs of the West Coast Navy

When opened, the hospital had 30 patient beds.[94] By the end of the first month of operation, all those beds were occupied, leading Surgeon Browne to write the bureau to request the opening of an additional ward for patients. The bureau promptly approved the request and, after seeking Browne's opinion about the advisability of supplying more expensive "fracture and invalid bedsteads," commented that "agreeably [sic] to your suggestion, [common] iron bedsteads will be employed."

Along with an expanding physical capacity, the staff began to grow to meet the demand of an increasing number of patients. On February 27, 1871, "Apothecary of the 1st Class" Mr. Joseph Anderson joined the hospital force,[95] and on March 8, Surgeon Browne wrote the Bureau of Medicine and Surgery to announce the appointment of Mrs. Elvira Baldwin "as an additional Nurse, with the assignment to duty as Matron of this Institution."[96] In his 1954 official history of the Mare Island Navy Yard, Arnold S. Lott states that Mrs. Baldwin was the first woman "in government employ" at the Navy base.[97] The Navy is a very conservative institution that values tradition, but I will argue several times in this book that the doctors at the naval hospital were innovators in this conservative culture. It was long a tradition that women and sailors don't mix well except in liberty ports or in the comfort of established families and homes. Accordingly, the Navy was late in accepting any role for women in the health-care establishment. That said, it was the Navy hospital that hired the first woman to work on Mare Island. Navy Yard historian

Four. A Hospital in Technological Transformation, 1871–1898

Sue Lemmon quoted from Mrs. Baldwin's March 1871 letter to a relative: "I have only to see that the attendants do their duty and see that the linen is properly cared for." She wrote that her annual salary was "only" $480, "although I have a prospect of having it raised soon."[98] I was unable to confirm this in my examination of hospital records, nor was I able to establish the term of Elvira Baldwin's pioneering role, though "one matron" at an annual salary of $480 is found listed in the estimates for employees for fiscal year ending June 30, 1874.[99]

By June, 45 beds had been set up, and in August, Surgeon G.W. Wood reported 60 available, and these were filled, prompting the harried doctor to reiterate the need for an assistant surgeon in a pointed letter back to the bureau. The need for additional medical help apparently was resolved, for the moment at least, with the arrival of Medical Inspector J.S. Dungan in the summer of 1872 to take charge of the hospital. Woods then reverted to the role of the assistant he had earlier requested.

In August 1872, Dungan submitted a budget to the bureau that called for a hospital medical staff that included (besides the medical inspector in charge and his assistant) the following:

- one apothecary at $1,000 per year
- one matron and four nurses at $480 each per year
- one engineer at $1,000
- one fireman at the gasworks at $750
- one fireman at the steam engine at $500
- one chief cook at $540
- one cook at $480
- one gardener at $600
- three washers at $480 each
- one watchman at $480 and one at $360
- three laborers at $420 each
- three messroom attendants at $250 each
- one stable keeper and driver at $480
- one messenger at $216

Part I—The Early Years

If approved, the total annual cost for these personnel would be $12,956.[100] Over the next couple of years, similar requests (though the matron was dropped) made their way to the bureau.

Two years after the hospital opened, the Panic of 1873 begot the "Long Depression" that lasted nearly a decade. It was a time of great social and economic upheaval: wages fell, unemployment reached 14 percent and businesses failed. Federal government revenue suffered as well, falling from its 1872 peak of more than $374 million to a low, in 1878, of almost $257 million, a drop of 31 percent! Navy expenditures plummeted an even more precipitous 41 percent.[101] Already in 1874, Medical Inspector Dungan was prompted to complain in a letter from June 1, 1874, "I earnestly urge you to approve the [staffing requested]. I beg to remind the Bureau that, while I have repeatedly asked for an increase of Employee's [sic], their number and the appropriation [for salaries], have both actually been reduced." (His annual budget for employees had dropped to $10,570.) Further, he grumbled, "I respectfully submit that the appropriation for the present fiscal year is inadequate to properly conduct this Institution and to take proper care of the Hospital grounds."[102] Dungan followed up on June 13 with a request that an additional medical officer be ordered to duty at the hospital.[103]

In August 1875, Medical Director Suddards reported that his staff included just one nurse, with an annual budget for his ten hospital employees of only $5338.20 (a very nearly 50 percent cut from 1874). He added,

> [You] will observe an Engineer and Fireman, whose collective pay amounts to $125.00 a month, or over one-fourth of the entire charge. These persons are engaged in the manufacture of gas, and the care & regulation of the supply of gas and water. Their duties are in no way connected with the care of the sick; and I would respectfully submit that in any comparison between the expenditures of this and other Hospitals, this fact should be carefully borne in mind.
>
> Again, I beg you to remark that a Purveyor is allowed, but no Apothecary. The duties of these two offices have been combined in one person. Is it so elsewhere? While it may answer in this special case, and be admitted as a temporary necessity; Any sudden change would subject us to great embarrassment.

Four. A Hospital in Technological Transformation, 1871–1898

Again, we have only one "nurse," for over forty (40) patients, with the possibility of large increase at any moment. I am sure you will agree with me that one Nurse cannot properly attend to this number of cases, scattered in separate wards, and in different parts of the building.

One "Watchman" and one "Messman" are also below our wants. As regards the latter, we have at present two officers, patients, and four Medical Officers on duty, all to be waited on and served by a single person. The mere statement is enough to show the absolute impossibility of the duties being performed.

We have no convalescents, whose services can be made available. Some four or five who had been made useful in various ways, were discharged just prior to my reporting for duty, through expiration of term of service.

In view therefore of the above-mentioned state … of help in this Hospital I would respectfully suggest the following additions to the list submitted.

One (1) Apothecary
One (1) Nurse
One (1) Washer
One (1) Watchman
One (1) Messman.[104]

Late in 1876, a Russian squadron put into the San Francisco Bay. At the time, tension between Russia and the Ottoman Empire over the czar's claim of protection over Orthodox Catholics in Ottoman territories looked like it might lead to war. The British and French appeared to be aligning themselves against the Russians, just as they had during the Crimean War a bit more than a decade earlier. In that contest, the powerful "allied" fleets combined to severely circumscribe the tactical effectiveness of the Russian Black Sea fleet and even moved against Russian ships in the North Pacific. In this case, the czar, in anticipation of a planned war against the Turks, sought to disperse his fleet. The San Francisco newspaper *Alta California*, in an editorial comment on February 7, 1877, put the matter thus: "The fleets of Russia's sloops of war are seeking American ports to be out of the way of the more formidable Navies of nations that might be her antagonists in case of a European war, or that they may be conveniently near some destined point of attack in case the peace of Europe and the world should be disturbed."[105] *Bayan* (18) [guns], flagship of the squadron, arrived in December; it was followed on January 18 by the steam-driven, iron-hulled schooner *Vostok*, which was soon

Part I—The Early Years

followed by the corvette *Tongas*, clippers *Abrek* and *Vsadnik* and the gunboats *Gornostai* and *Japonetz*.[106]

The arrival of several hundred Russian sailors at Mare Island soon showed its impact on the hospital. On January 16, 1877, Hospital Commander Browne wrote to the bureau, "I have to inform the Bureau that on the 30th ult [previous month, in this case, December], by order of Rear Admiral Jno. Rodgers, Commandant, two of the crew of the Russian Flag Ship 'Bayan' were received at this institution for treatment & subsistence, where they now remain." Twelve days later, Browne noted that his patient load was now 49, including no fewer than 14—1 officer, 13 men—from the Russian fleet. He added,

> As the Russian fleet is to be increased by the addition of three other vessels, making a total of nine, & will continue here for some time, it is probable a large number of their sick will be sent to the Hospital.... I am aware that the Bureau is compelled to exercise unusual economy in its expenditures, yet in view of the present requirements, which are likely to be increased, I deem it my duty to make this representation, that the Bureau, if possible, may be pleased to authorize the appointment of two mess room attendants at $25 currency, each, per month.[107]

In a February 12 update, Browne stated that 1 Russian officer and 14 men remained in hospital "with a probability of further addition," and he requested "instructions concerning the payment of the cost of maintenance, i.e., if each man shall be charged thirty cents and each officer sixty cents a day."[108]

Even though Russian armies were active on many fronts in the Balkans and Caucasus, apparently the anticipated allied naval "interference" was not forthcoming, so the Russian squadron debarked in May, prompting Browne to remark,

> The Russian Fleet having departed, I have, in accordance with the instructions contained in your letter of February 7th, this day discharged the mess room attendant, who was paid on bill similar to the extra employe's [sic]. I regret the loss of the said attendant, for although the emergency that occasioned his appointment has passed, yet his services would obviate the necessity of substituting convalescents, none of whom are [sic] reliable or constant. Two of the Russian sick, wholly incurable, remain in the hospital, & I am uninformed as to their intended disposition, no notification

Four. A Hospital in Technological Transformation, 1871–1898

having been received as to the expected or desired continuance at this institution.[109]

One gets the impression that communication between the Russian admiral and the medical officer in charge was less than effective, despite Browne's attendance at such social events as the "brilliant assemblage" of officers and civilians who attended a "matinee" dance hosted by Russian Admiral Pousino on March 5![110]

However, 1876 appears to have seen the nadir of funding for hospital personnel. A circular from the chief of the bureau (William Grier) to Browne in November 1877 told him that the Secretary of the Navy himself had directed, in a new policy, that apothecaries assigned to naval hospitals, once they signed a contract to the effect, would henceforth be paid from "pay of the Navy" money, rather than hospital budgets. "The amount thus saved" in this transfer of pay responsibility, the Bureau directed, could then be applied for paying such additional staff or increasing the pay of current staff, as the surgeon in charge might decide.

Medical Inspector Browne submitted a budget calling for $6,600 (including two nurses) for fiscal year 1879. This number rose to $7,800 (and three nurses) the following year. As late as 1881, Medical Inspector Peck, Browne's successor, was moved to write,

> At the commencement of a new fiscal year I desire to call the attention of the Bureau to the number, pay, and ratings of the civil employes of this Hospital, and to urge some changes which seem to be needed.
> The constantly higher rate of wages in California as compared with the Eastern States makes it impossible to hire suitable men to fill the present ratings at the wages allowed by the Bureau. Many of those employed during the past year have proved unsatisfactory, some for dissolute habits, while others have become discontented with their lot, and have found a more remunerative field of labor. Since August 1st, 1880, when the present schedule of pay went into effect, as ordered by the Bureau, twenty employes in the various departments have been discharged—three for misconduct, the others at their own request. At the end of the last Quarter, the Chief Nurse, who has served in the Hospital ever since it was established, left in order to obtain more pay, and the place of Asst. Nurse has been filled during the twelvemonth by seven different persons. The comparative isolation of this Hospital also tends to make vacancies, as the difficulty of crossing the strait

Part I—The Early Years

to Vallejo, a mile distant, interferes to prevent those who incline to seek recreation there, while it also deters those who might seek employment.

The necessity of a larger number of employes here than some other Hospital arises from the fact, due to the peculiarities of soil, climate, etc., that the grounds, outbuildings, and fences in close proximity to the Hospital require attention throughout the year. These considerations induce me to appeal for a larger monthly allowance for the civil list of this institution in order to secure faithful men in the future, and I trust that the Bureau will authorize the ratings and pay of the enclosed list, as a basis for the current fiscal year. At present rates of pay it is impossible to procure a competent cook. The Driver is, of necessity, absent from the stable a considerable part of the time, as he not only drives the ambulance, but performs all the work of transportation for the Hospital. The Hostler assists in the care of the Stable and the Stock, Driving, milking, cleaning, etc.—The wear and tear of the buildings and fences require the constant services of a Carpenter. The total monthly pay proposed is five hundred ($500.00) dollars [or $6,000 annually, still no higher than previous budgets].[111]

Austerity was the rule of the day, however, and Surgeon General Wales replied allowing only $400 per month for payment of employees, adding, "[This] sum is all the appropriation for [the employee budget] will admit of for that [Mare Island] hospital, for the current fiscal year."[112] This is not the first time or the last that we will read of the higher cost of labor in California. Medical Inspector Peck put the matter most directly in his letter to the bureau on September 26, 1882:

The small amount allotted for the current expenses of the hospital leads me to refer once more to the difficulty of keeping the Hospital and its surroundings in a proper state of neatness; it is indeed impossible to do so. The grounds are large, and considerable labor is required to keep merely the roads and walks immediately about the house in order; still, we have no gardener and not even a laborer for this duty. With a list of sick which rose as high as fifty during the last quarter, we have but one nurse, and he is so scantily paid that he is liable to leave at any time.

Two cooks are absolutely needed for the prompt and suitable preparation of food. We are unable to hire a fireman; hence waste of material from inefficient firing, together with risk to boilers and damage to machinery, as the Engineer, who has charge of all gas and water apparatus as well as the steam pumps and boilers must divide his time among his various duties and cannot give exclusive attention to any one of them.

It is impossible for the one launderer to do all the work of the Hospital laundry in a proper manner. A carpenter (or general utility man) is needed

Four. A Hospital in Technological Transformation, 1871–1898

imperatively in an institution such as this, where no day passes without the occurrence of something, within doors, or without, requiring repair.

As for the need for a Driver, it will be remembered that our daily supplies all come from Vallejo and are delivered at the ferry more than a mile from the Hospital, from which place we have to transport them in the Hospital wagon.

I trust it will be clear from the above & from what I have written previously, at various times, that the estimate—as per schedule—of fifteen employees is not excessive. With the present allowance of one hundred and eighty-four dollars per month only six employes [sic] can be secured.

Peck's proposed schedule of pay of civil employees for fiscal year 1883–4 was $6,000. This would provide a staff of

1 Engine-tender per month	$60
1 Fireman	$30
1 Chief Cook	$40
1 Assistant Cook	$20
1 Driver	$35
1 Stableman	$30
2 Launderers $30 and $25	$55
1 Messroom Attendant	$30
1 Gardener	$35
1 Carpenter	$35
2 Nurses, each $35	$70
2 Laborers, each $30	$60[113]

In August, Peck wrote the bureau to request the hire of a messman to fill in while his nurse was himself a patient. He added that the nurse was soon to be discharged from the Navy and that he desired to hire him on as a civilian, "as he is thoroughly competent, and it is necessary that we should have one nurse, at least."[114]

In a telegram of August 10, the employee budget was reduced to $184 per month, representing a reduction of more than 50 percent from the reduced budget offered two years before. In July 1884, the bureau increased total employee pay to $200 a month.[115]

There the matter apparently lay until October 1886, when Gihon wrote Bureau Chief Francis Gunnell,

Part I—The Early Years

> There is but one nurse attached to this Hospital, who is required to care for all the patients in the two wards, which are at the extreme opposite ends of the building. He is on duty every day from 6 a.m. to 9 p.m., without relief.
>
> There is a night watchman (who is required on account of the greater danger from fire on this island—through the scarcity of water) who also attends to such patients as may require assistance after 9 p.m.
>
> The number of very sick is now, however, so great that the one nurse is insufficient: he is breaking down; and will soon himself become ill if not relieved. I have, accordingly, to recommend the appointment of an additional nurse at Twenty Dollars a month pay, and am, fortunately, able to secure the services of a thoroughly competent nurse, very highly recommended by Surgeon Woolverton. It is impossible to re-arrange the list of employes, who are now receiving minimum pay and not one of whom can be dispensed with, without serious interference with the duties of the Hospital. Even with these allowed employes, it would be impossible to continue the necessary work of the Hospital without the aid of convalescent patients, as assistant to the Engineer, as messenger and mail carrier, as orderlies at the front door, and as helpers about the grounds and in the building.[116]

Five days later, Gihon wrote the bureau to complain that with the onset of winter weather, hallway temperatures had dropped to 53°, obligating him to start up the steam-heating apparatus. His engineer informed him that a fireroom watch would be necessary but that he had no one available for the task, including convalescents. He went on,

> The Engineer further objects to the additional labor of watching the large number of steam-heaters, distributed on the several floors throughout the building, repairing steam pipes and valves and performing other machinist work upon his present rate of pay (forty dollars). The pay of ordinary firemen on the river-steamboats is fifty dollars and upwards and I have accordingly to represent the urgent necessity for an increased allowance of thirty-five dollars [totaling $75] per month for the engineer's force at this Hospital.[117]

He added a listing of his staff, responsible for an institution caring for around 40 patients, to be an engineer (at $40 a month), stableman ($25), nurse ($25), messman ($25), night watchman ($20—he cared for patients when the nurse was not on duty, namely from 9:00 p.m. to 6:00 a.m., seven days a week), laborer ($20), cook ($30), assistant cook ($20) and scrubber ($20). Sick officers paid their own servants for room cleaning, assistance with meals and the like. Surgeon General Gunnell apparently did not reply to these and other requests

Four. A Hospital in Technological Transformation, 1871–1898

for additional staff, and subsequent correspondence from Gihon mentioned work around the hospital, especially on the grounds, being performed by convalescent patients.

The next correspondence around staffing appeared in 1893, when Medical Inspector G.W. Woods wrote,[118]

> I would respectfully present for your consideration the following extract from my last Annual Report, deeming it to be of such importance that it should not fail of being brought to your special attention on assuming the duties of Surgeon-General, so that if it meets with your favorable consideration, the requisite increase in appropriation may be demanded from the next Congress, should that be necessary....
>
> Again, two nurses are entirely inadequate to the proper care and attention of three wards with an average of 45 patients, and to perform, also, the special services required by sick officers; while $25 per month will not secure in California, a man of pronounced ability, and integrity, to remain contentedly in such a position save under exceptional circumstances....
>
> Lastly during the Winter, an additional fireman should be employed. At present the steam is kept up from 6:30 a.m. to 8:30 p.m. as a necessity for even moderate comfort, and the duty is of such a character that a relief for the regular fireman is reluctantly secured from amongst the convalescent patients who may belong to the engineer force, and be sufficiently strong for such service....
>
> The following schedule of employe's [sic], with pay in accordance to their duties, and the customary rates of wages on the Pacific coast is respectfully submitted:

		(Rate of pay at Navy Yard)
Apothecary	$1000 per year	
Engineer	$75 per month	Present pay, $50
Carpenter	45 " "	" " 35
Cook	35	30
Asst Cook	25	20
Gardener	40	35
Driver	40	35
Stableman	30	25
Nurses (30) each	30	25 each (2)
Scrubber	30	25
Messman	30	25
Laborer	30	25
Firemen (2) each	30	25
Master-at-arms	30	25

Part I—The Early Years

Once again, the higher cost of workers in California is apparent, and I find it interesting that the gardener is paid more than the nurses.

And there, the staffing matter stood until the end of the decade.

Hospital Routine Barely Interrupted

Despite the various matters concerning the physical plant and staffing, the routine of the hospital went on. The patients needed to be fed, and the staff maintained a herd of cows and gardens in addition to purchasing from local grocers. Medicines needed to be procured and surgical instruments provided.

One priority was to create a proper medical library. In 1875, Suddards put it this way:

> I respectfully beg to call your attention to the urgent want of a Medical Library at this Hospital. In looking over the letter-book, I find that Dr Dungan sent to the Bureau under date of Nov 19th 1874, a list of books then on the shelves. Many even of those are the private property of Surgeon Wm. E. Taylor now attached to the Yard. There have been no additions since that date. As the assistants at Hospitals are generally young men entitled to an examination for promotion, it occurs to me that a properly & well selected Library of Books of Standard Merit, might be an inducement to them to increased application. Leaving the matter to your good judgment and direction.[119]

The bureau's response wasn't immediate, but by 1880, fairly regular, cryptic acknowledgments for such books as "Keyes' 'Venereal Diseases'" or "Guttman on Physical Diagnosis" and even "Munde on Minor Surgical Gynecology" (remember this was an all-male environment of practice) appear in correspondence back to the bureau. "MacCormac on Antiseptic Surgery" arrived in November of that year.[120]

As manifested by the receipt of these books, medicine and surgery had seen significant scientific advances over the last quarter of the century. The discovery of X-ray had revolutionized the diagnosis of such diseases as tuberculosis and pneumonia. An emerging understanding of how the body works (physiology) and the nature of diseases (pathology) led to an increasing dependence on the medical laboratory. Surgery, though still fraught, was benefiting from better understanding of anatomy and refinements in anesthesia. While antibiotics were yet to be discovered, the role of bacteria in the spread and cause of diseases like cholera, tuberculosis and syphilis led to more effective means of prevention through public health interventions. That the treatment of disease was becoming more "evidence based" is well represented by the thinking of the famed Johns Hopkins professor of medicine William Osler, who acknowledged in a 1909 speech to the Ontario (Canada) Medical Association, "As an enemy to indiscriminate drugging, I have often been branded as a therapeutic nihilist.... I bore this reproach cheerfully, coming, as I knew it did, from men who did not appreciate the difference between the giving of medicine and the treatment of disease."[121]

Finally, a House for the Hospital Commander

A year and a half after the hospital opened, we learn from Dungan's estimates for repairs and improvements of a need for a house for the senior doctor (at a cost of $28,000), with this curt comment: "I recommend the erection of a house for the Medical Officer in Charge of the Hospital which shall correspond in style with the Hospital, which is a handsome structure," adding, "I earnestly request you to ask for appropriations for [this]."[122] He repeated this request in identical terms in 1872.[123]

There the matter lay until October 1876, when Browne, in his annual estimate of improvements needed, wrote,

> Surgeon's House. As no appartments [sic] are provided in the Hospital for the residence of the Surgeon in charge, it is presumed that the Department intends to erect a house for the Surgeon, in proximity to the institution. To the southwest of the Hospital, and separated from it by a ravine, upon a Commanding Eminence, with protecting hills in the rear, is the site recommended for this purpose. The grounds possess a natural beauty and could with ease and economy be connected with the Hospital grounds by a light bridge crossing the ravine, thereby rendering the situation accessible and picturesque. For the Surgeon's house, outbuildings, fences, and cistern, the estimated cost is $28,000.[124]

Part I—The Early Years

Similar requests were made almost annually thereafter, with estimated costs ranging as low as $20,000. Browne's comment is somewhat misleading because the chief doctor and his family actually lived in an apartment on the hospital second floor.[125] Although not in the original hospital design, the expediency was apparently settled on from the first days of hospital operation.

Gihon fully described the situation in a September 12, 1888, letter to the chief of the bureau:

> In anticipation of my transfer to other duty, which is assurance that no consideration of personal comfort or convenience are herein involved, I try to again represent to the Bureau, the very urgent need of quarters for the Medical Director in Charge of this hospital outside the Hospital itself.
>
> The accompanying plan [absent in the record] represents the considerable portion of the second floor of the building occupied by the Medical Director in Charge and which the proper seclusion of the family of this officer will not permit to be encroached upon. These apartments are manifestly not well adapted for occupancy by a family comprising female members, children, guests and women servants. The approach to this suite of rooms is by the main stairway, for children and servants as well as others, unless they are permitted to use a side stairway in common with patients and employes. The very grave objection to allowing children and female domestics to have access to the very interior of an institution of this character does not require argument.
>
> The dining-room of the Medical Director in Charge is a portion of Ward 4, directly over Ward 1, and social entertainments obligatory upon this officer necessarily disturb the patients immediately beneath, especially after 9 p.m., when the lights in the wards are extinguished. The room occupied as a parlor, which is only ten feet wide and the adjoining sitting room and chamber, which are but twenty inches [*sic?*] wide, are of inadequate size for these purposes, while they could conveniently serve for sick quarters for individual occupants.
>
> The assistant medical officers are now quartered on the first floor, where they occupy rooms that might properly be diverted to other purposes. The office of the Medical Director in Charge is a small apartment, having an unencumbered floor space, less than six feet wide by nine feet long, partitioned off from the dispensary, of which it should be a part. The "officer of the day" has no office apart from the apothecary, and there is no room which can be used by visitors to enlisted patients, nor one in which religious services may be held, when these may be required. The abandonment of the rooms now occupied by the Medical Director will not only provide quarters on the second floor for a proper complement of assistant medical officers, which is not now possible, as well as for sick officers, but will enable

Four. A Hospital in Technological Transformation, 1871–1898

the apartments of the first floor to be used for the public purposes above indicated.

The grounds within the limits of the Hospital reservation fortunately furnish admirable sites for a residence for the Medical Officer in Charge. Out of these, "A" on the accompanying plan is on the slope of a hill in the south course of the reservation; a second, "B" on the plan, and <u>in my opinion more desirable location</u> [underlining mine], is in the opposite direction, near the western boundary of the grounds on the side facing the Marine Barracks, north-west from the Hospital, behind the bridge now bordering the plank-walk from the Navy-Yard. A house can be erected on the slope of the hill at this spot, affording a view of San Pablo Bay in the rear, as well as of the Navy-Yard, and, Vallejo and its surrounding in front. This site is convenient to the stables, accessible from the Navy-Yard, and commands the direct approaches to the Hospital. The other is distant in all these respects, and is, further, separated from the elevation in which the Hospital stands by a deep gulley.

A cottage-built dwelling at the site recommended, capacious enough for a family however large, with all the necessary conveniences, and arrangements of modern life, can be erected <u>for less than $18,000</u>, including all the expenses of connections with the Hospital system of water supply, steam heating, gas-lighting, sewerage and drainage.

He closed:

> I need not remind the Bureau that all the Naval Hospitals, except the small establishment at Washington, have separate houses for the families of the Medical Officers in Charge, and that the conditions, which make this so necessary at Boston, New York, Philadelphia, and Norfolk, exist in even greater degree at this the only Naval Hospital on this coast, for both the extensive Pacific and Asiatic Stations.[126]

The Surgeon General sent this report up the chain of command in his statistical report on the health of the Navy, dated October 25, 1888:

> During the past two years this hospital has had extensive repairs and is now in excellent condition. The Bureau has frequently called attention to the urgent need of separate quarters for the Medical Officer in Charge. In their absence he is obliged to occupy rooms intended for the junior medical officers and a ward which has never been used for patients. [He then uses arguments submitted by Gihon.] ... For the purposes of removing the embarrassment, estimates are submitted for building a house for the Medical Director at a cost of $20,000, including all the expenses of connections with the hospital system of water supply, heating, gas lighting, sewerage and drainage, which it is hoped will meet your approval.[127]

Part I—The Early Years

A year later, Browne wrote to the Secretary of the Navy,

At other stations the medical officer in charge has quarters apart from the hospital. At Mare Island he is compelled to occupy a ward as there is no house, and this ward is needed for the accommodation of the sick. The hospital receives patients from the Pacific and Asiatic Stations, and is second in importance to the hospital in Brooklyn. In my annual report of last year attention was called to the urgency for providing such quarters, and it will be renewed in the report for the present year. Permit me to state that there is reason to believe the appropriation will be made by the next Congress if so, it would be desirable to determine the site for the house that no unnecessary delay might occur.[128]

A year later, Browne wrote in his annual report,

This hospital was built in 1869–'70. Since that time in eight annual reports of this Bureau attention has been called to the urgent need of separate quarters for the medical officer in charge. The architect did not provide for the residence of this officer within the building. At the hospitals on the Atlantic coast, except Washington, houses are provided for such officers, and their families. There are no houses at Mare Island that can be rented. The medical director is compelled to occupy rooms intended for a junior medical officer, and a ward which has never been used for the sick. The junior medical officers have rooms on the first floor which could be put to public use, if the medical director resided without the building. With the increasing demand for space for accommodating patients this arrangement causes great inconvenience. The hospital is second in importance to that at Brooklyn. Many patients are sent from the Pacific and Asiatic stations for treatment or discharge. Some by reason of advanced age are unfit for further service, and although entitled to the privileges of the Naval Home are unwilling to exchange the advantages of the climate for the severer one of the east; others whose homes are in the vicinity wish to remain in California. A number of paralytics and infirm seamen and marines, constantly increasing, from causes incident to the service, for whom provision should be made for their subsistence and caretaking, thereby avoiding the crowded condition of the Naval Home at Philadelphia, and the expense of transfer thereto. The vacation of the ward now occupied by the medical director in charge would afford facilities for this purpose which would probably suffice for years.

In view of removing the embarrassment, estimates are submitted for building a house for the medical director at a cost of $15,500 including all expenses of connections with the hospital system of water supply, heating, lighting, sewerage and drainage, for which your approval is earnestly solicited.[129]

In April 1890, Browne followed this up with a letter to the Honorable W.B. Allison, chairman of the Senate Committee on

Four. A Hospital in Technological Transformation, 1871–1898

Appropriations, requesting an appropriation of $15,500 for a medical director's residence, and he used the same arguments: that the hospital was the only one on the West Coast and thus as important or more important than the several East Coast naval hospitals that provided such quarters.[130]

Finally, the breakthrough happened. The Digest of Naval Appropriations for the Fiscal Year 1892 arrived at the bureau. The entry on page 21: "For construction of a residence for the medical director in charge of naval hospital at Mare Island, California, in full for all expenses of erecting and making necessary improvements about the grounds, fifteen thousand five hundred dollars."[131]

> Navy Department, Bureau of Medicine and Surgery, Washington, D.C., September 23rd, 1891. Sealed proposals, in duplicate, are hereby invited and will be received at this office until Monday, November 2nd, 1891, at 11 a.m., at which time and place they will be publicly opened in the presence of attending bidders, for building a residence for the Medical Director of Naval Hospital, at the Navy Yard, Mare Island, California, in accordance with the plans and specifications which may be seen at the Naval Hospital, Mare Island, California.[132]

Architectural drawings of a lovely (described at the time as "colonial" style) home of modest proportions, were produced by Treasury Department architect Ervin S. Hubbard.[133]

From here, things moved pretty quickly: a contract was signed with J.B. McKenzie of Benicia, California, at the end of November, and after a brief delay due "to some informality," the contractor received the go-ahead on January 5, 1893. Early on, the site for the home, on a knoll to the west and south of the hospital, was found to be too rocky for ploughing. Trenching and blasting were required to remove ground for the cellar. It being the rainy season, weather-related delays were inevitable. As construction proceeded, Surgeon General Browne made the decision to provide both electrical and gas lighting. Supervising Engineer Maxson requested the provision for light switches, including "three way switches, so that the lights (in upstairs and downstairs hallways) can be turned on and off from either the first or second story, etc.—[which] would

Part I—The Early Years

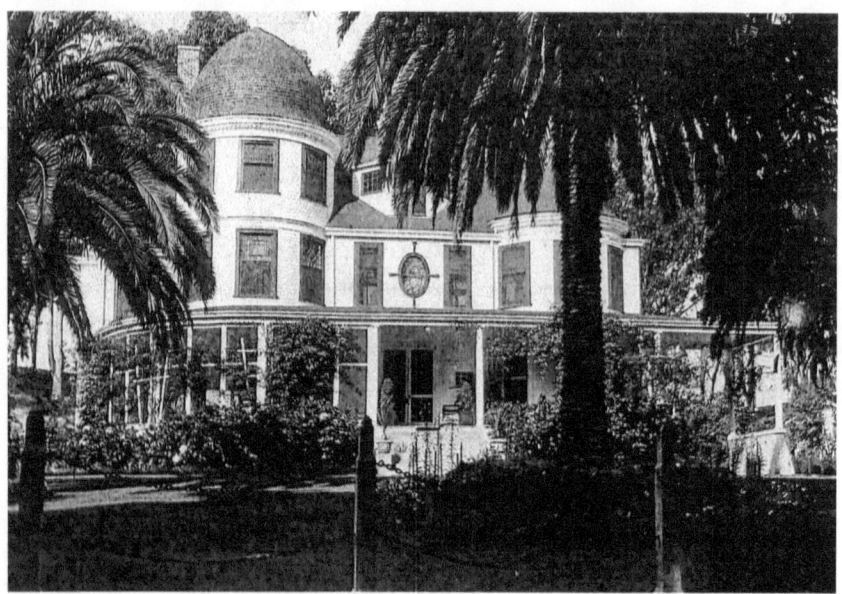

Hospital commander's home, Mare Island, California. Date and source uncertain. Mare Island Historic Park Foundation, Vallejo, California.

materially increase the convenience and use of the electric lights when they are installed, and would prevent the defacement of the walls when introducing switches after the building is finished." This Browne approved, for an additional cost of $35.[134] On November 15, with external grading and steam, water, gas and drain connections completed and tested, Engineer Maxson declared the house and grounds ready for occupancy. Total payments to the contractor added up to $14,910. Medical Inspector G.W. Woods, who had been at the Mare Island hospital soon after it opened in 1871, became the first resident in what would be home for hospital commanders for the next 80 years.[135]

A Premonition

Local newspapers (*Sacramento Daily Union* and *San Francisco Morning Call*) reported a severe earthquake on April 19. With an

Four. A Hospital in Technological Transformation, 1871–1898

epicenter estimated to be in Vacaville, about 22 miles distant to the east, damage was fortunately light. Although underreported by the *Daily Union*—"a brick was shaken out of the gable end of a sawmill"—Woods wrote in May to request "that a sum of $28.96 be transferred to the Department of Yards and Docks for labor to be performed in repairing chimneys on the roof of the Hospital, recently damaged by earthquakes."[136]

Then on March 31, 1898, the Secretary of the Navy received this telegram from Captain of the Navy Yard Henry Glass ("Commanding"): "Very heavy earthquake last night 11:45 doing great damage saw mill and paint shop C & R. Entirely destroyed building sixty nine, badly damaged hospital and buildings numbers one to fourteen all damaged more or less severely ... no injury of any kind to persons." Another telegram from Glass arrived at the Surgeon General's office at 3:15 p.m.: "Hospital building seriously damaged by earthquake last night survey ordered request authority to make some immediate repairs," to which the bureau replied by telegraph, "Repairs essential to immediate safety authorized." And on April 4, "Forward by telegraph to Bureau as soon as possible estimated cost to permanently repair property under Bureau M[edicine] & S[urgery], damaged by earthquake," and on April 7, "Telegraph immediately rough estimate of cost to permanently repair property,"[137] to which Navy Yard Commandant W.A. Kirkland telegraphed on April 7, "Board survey.... Will finish examination tomorrow. Hospital building probably condemned better ask for enough money to build steel framed hospital."[138]

The damage was indeed severe. The *San Francisco Call* on April 1 reported,

> Where the seismic force wrought its greatest harm was at the Navy Hospital, a massive building of brick, standing on the north slope of a hill on the southern end [*sic*] of the island. Originally the building cost $175,000 [*sic*]. It was built in the most solid manner, and the thickness of its walls can be measured in feet. It has stood twenty-nine years, but last night's shake has split it in a hundred different directions, and daylight filters through some of the rents in its walls.[139]

Part I—The Early Years

On April 8, Commandant Kirkland wired, "Board survey recommends condemnation hospital building. Estimates can be based only on plans adopted by Bureau," to which the bureau responded the same day, "Will hospital building be safe for inmates when present repairs are completed?" The next day, Kirkland telegrammed, "No repairs being made. All work has been tearing down chimneys and plaster likely to fall immediately in case repairs were attempted the building must be unoccupied."[140] Two days later, on April 11, the Surgeon General wrote to the Secretary of the Navy,

> I have the honor to request that an appropriation of one hundred thousand dollars ($100,000) may be asked for, to be included in the Naval Appropriation Bill now pending, for tearing down and removing present Naval Hospital building and appendages recently destroyed by earthquake at Navy Yard, Mare Island, California, and erecting a new Naval Hospital and appendages at that place. The appropriation to be immediately available.
>
> The original cost of the present Hospital was one hundred and twenty-seven thousand dollars ($127,000). It accommodates ninety patients and has been filled to its utmost capacity. It is proposed to erect in its stead a wooden building of about the same capacity, with improvements in construction and adaptation in accordance with modern hospital requirements.

He added, importantly, "I am informed by the Colonel Commandant of the Marine Corps that the patients from the Hospital have been temporarily transferred to the Marine Barracks."[141]

FIVE

Early 20th Century

On April 11, 1898, the medical inspector in charge of the hospital, G.P. Bradley, submitted his formal report on the earthquake in which, first, he detailed the urgent transfer of enlisted patients to the second story of one wing of the nearby Marine barracks.[12] Hospitalized officers were to be cared for in USS *Pensacola*, then present at the Navy Yard. Bradley detailed the need for a very prompt construction of a new hospital. In support of his request, he cited the "insanitary" nature of the barracks, the remoteness of latrine facilities, the need for an adequate food preparation facility nearby, and the lack of an adequate operating room. He specifically ventured the recommendation for an expanded facility of 100 beds be constructed, adding, "If a thoroughly modern and efficient hospital is to be erected, I would observe that present modes of steel construction have been tested in this region and found to be quite secure from earthquake shocks, ... and would ... assure such a building at a reasonable, and in the end, economical, price."[3]

Nine days later, Surgeon General Van Reypen, replying to a verbal request from the Honorable Joseph G. Cannon, chairman of the House Committee on Appropriations, made his request for $100,000 for removing the old hospital and placing a new one "on the present site, the only one available." Citing the growth of the Navy, the steady receipt of patients from ships of Pacific and Asiatic squadrons, and from naval hospitals at Sitka, Alaska, and Yokohama, Japan, as well as from other West Coast Navy stations and the Coast Survey and Fish Commission, he urged the new facility be of at least 100 beds.[4] The appropriations were duly approved on May 4, 1898.

Part I—The Early Years

While the earthquake drama and its aftermath on Mare Island was taking place, an even larger event was engaging the attention of the folks in Washington, D.C. A month and a half before the earthquake struck Mare Island, the USS *Maine* blew up in Havana Harbor in Cuba. While subsequent investigations have suggested that some sort of internal explosion sunk the ship, an investigation conducted by Navy officials—the "Sampson Board"—within days after the explosion concluded that a mine had been the culprit. Anti-Spanish sentiment—already running high in the United States because of Spanish suppression of a Cuban independence movement, and encouraged by Hearst- and Pulitzer-owned newspapers—leaped to fever pitch. A slow-rolling movement developed that led ultimately to the Spanish-American War. This was to have major impact on the naval hospital.

On May 23, Surgeon General Van Reypen had a conversation with D.C. architect W.M. Poindexter, the subject being the creation of plans for a new hospital at Mare Island. The next day, Van Reypen informed the Secretary of the Navy that he intended to engage Mr. Poindexter "to prepare plans, specifications, and detail drawings for the construction and finishing of building or buildings ... for three and one half (3–½) per centum on the amount of the contract price for the completed works, this being the usual and proper charge endorsed by the American Institute of Architects."[5] Meanwhile, the Surgeon General's Office and the Colonel Commandant of the Marine Corps made arrangements that the bureau would pay one-third of the expense for water and electric lights at the Marine Corps barracks for the period that the building served as a temporary hospital facility.[6] When, on June 29, California senator George C. Perkins made inquiry as to when bids were to be sought (his letter was addressed to the "Supervising Surgeon-General, Marine [now Public] Hospital Service" and forwarded to the bureau), Van Reypen replied that the advertisements would likely appear in the *Government Advertiser* and "probably in Vallejo and San Francisco" most likely in early August 1898.[7]

In a "Requisition for Advertising," dated August 26, Surgeon

Five. Early 20th Century

General Van Reypen requested approval to seek bids "for tearing down and removing present Naval Hospital building, and for erection and completion of a new naval Hospital, at the U.S. Navy Yard, Mare Island, Cal. Plans, specifications and blank forms of proposal can be had upon application to the Naval Hospital ... where any additional information can be obtained."[8]

In the same report, Van Reypen noted that Congress, responding to an urgent appeal for funding for a replacement for the earthquake-damaged structure, had duly appropriated funding "for tearing down and removing present naval hospital building ... recently destroyed by earthquake ... and erecting a new naval hospital and appendages at that place, to be immediately available, one hundred thousand dollars." He went on,

> As soon as the appropriation became available ... Mr William M Poindexter, an architect of this city [D.C.], was authorized to prepare plans, specifications and detail drawings for the new naval hospital building. The work was advertised for on September 1, 1898, and bids for the same will be opened in this Bureau at 1 p.m., October 12, 1898. The new hospital will be constructed on the foundation walls of the old building, so far as the old work will conform to the new conditions and requirements. The plans and specifications of the new building provide for a generous increase of area for administrative departments of the hospital on the first and second stories, and for suites of rooms (each suite consisting of a parlor, bed-room, bath-room and water closet) for sick officers on the third floor. The rear extension of the hospital provides ample accommodation for the kitchen, offices and mess halls on the first floor; etherizing [we would say "preoperative preparation" today], operation and recovery rooms, dispensary and chapel on the second floor; and bedrooms for the use of attendants on the third floor. The basement of the entire building will be used for no other purposes than for general storage, water-closets, and one large room for a men's smoking-room.[9]

He went on to describe the hospital as accommodating four wards of 20 beds each (expandable to double this capacity in an emergency), with ventilating ducts beneath each bed by which "foul air will be drawn from the wards by exhaust fans," and "in every department of the proposed building particular attention has been bestowed on all sanitary matters and appliances, and to the most approved methods of heating, ventilating and electric wiring." He added that an electric elevator was to be provided and noted that this

Part I—The Early Years

time, the building would be "of wood frame construction, of a most substantial character, and the exterior and interior finish of California redwood."[10]

It is interesting to observe that as of this writing, this structure, designated "H-1" in the Mare Island Naval Hospital complex, has survived several large earthquakes—the most substantial ones being in 1906 (7.7 intensity), 1957 (5.3), 1969 (5.6 and 5.7) and 2014 (6.0)—without substantial damage.

"NAVAL HOSPITAL AT MARE ISLAND," blared a page 12 headline in the September 3, 1898, *San Francisco Call*. "Plans for a Very Fine Structure TO BE THE BEST ON THE COAST, California Redwood with Stone Foundation [*sic*], Anticipating a Recurrence of Earthquake, the Authorities Have Taken Every Precaution."[11]

The bids were duly opened, and the lowest bidder, at $71,000, was one John J. Flanagan. The bureau telegraphed, "What sort of man is Flanagan. Wire reply." There followed quite a flurry of telegraph traffic about the low bidder, as he seemed to be known only as a journeyman stonecutter. The second lowest bidder, contractor Andrew Dahlberg, even weighed in by letter on the 15th:

> Believing I am the lowest legal bidder for the proposed Naval Hospital at Mare Island, I write to say if your Department awards me the contract I am ready to qualify in stipulated Bond & press the work with all haste consistent with proper caution to insure good work.... This man Flanigan was brought forward today after various efforts to locate him & induced to join the Builders Association. He is entirely unknown among the contractors on this coast—and had been engaged here as a journey man stone cutter. I feel satisfied when the Department are fully acquainted with the facts in the case, and ther [*sic*] knowledge of said Flannigan's noncompliance with the Law governing.... Contracts they will in justice to me award me the contract for construction of said Naval Hospital at Mare Island, Cal.

Medical Inspector Bradley made a trip to San Francisco to investigate the situation on October 28. His conclusion: Flanagan was neither capable nor competent to fulfill the contract. After consulting with Navy lawyers and receiving confirmation that Dahlberg was a respectable and able contractor, the bureau let the bid to him on November 4. Dahlberg's bid, at $72,441.00, was close enough to

Five. Early 20th Century

Flanagan's of $71,000. The Surgeon General also received, on October 29, a letter from contractor Dennis Jordan:

> Seeing by the specifications of the new Naval Hospital at Mare Island, that you have the appointing of a superintendent to take charge of its construction, I take the liberty of addressing you and respectfully request you to appoint me.... As I was the contractor for the present building, I would take pleasure in having charge of its reconstruction.

Perhaps recalling the legion of plumbing difficulties in the "present building," the Surgeon General replied, "You are informed that the Superintendent of construction, referred to in the specifications for the New Naval Hospital at Mare Island, Cal., will be detailed from the Corps of Engineers, U.S. Navy."

The contract was duly prepared on November 4. An embarrassed Dahlberg telegraphed on November 17 that due to a clerical error, the wrong number was written on his bid, which was intended to be $82,741. The Judge Advocate General weighed in: "[The] contract should be made out from the written words and not the figures. If you refuse to sign the contract as made out, return it to the Bureau. Contract will be awarded to another, and your sureties will be held for the difference." The contractor "folded": the hospital commander reported on December 21 that "Mr A. Dahlberg commenced the work of tearing down the condemned hospital building on the 19th instant, and that the old building was entirely vacated yesterday."[12]

From then, work proceeded apace. On February 4, 1899, Engineer Hollyday reported that 30 to 37 men were working on the project, that 700 loads of broken brick and mortar had been removed from the site, excavation for the new wing "practically completed" and 113,000 old bricks had been cleaned for reuse. He added, "The corner stone of the old hospital has been found embedded in the wall above the water table at the north-east corner, it was delivered sealed to Medical Inspector G.P. Bradley." A week later, Hollyday wrote to point out that the original plans called for installation of fittings for gas lighting in the hospital and pointed out that the gas plant on the island had long been torn down and gas mains pulled up and that the Navy electricity generating plant was "being constantly increased

Part I—The Early Years

in capacity." The bureau replied, "After careful consideration of the matter, [we] have decided to have the gas-fittings installed in the hospital, as called for in by the specifications and the terms of the contract." Nevertheless, electrical conduit men were on the job on May 20, along with "33 carpenters, 4 plumbers and gasfitters, 6 laborers and 2 teamsters." The work continued, though at a pace sometimes too slow for the taste of the supervising engineer, now Stanford. That said, by the end of July, the building was entirely framed in and the roofs nearly completed.

A glitch occurred as the interior was being plastered in that the material quickly developed cracks and began to peel off the ceilings and walls as it dried. The plasterers union (Golden Gate Lodge No. 1, Plasterers of San Francisco International Union 118) even weighed in, blaming the (non-union?) plasterer subcontractor,[13] but Superintendent of Construction Sanford concluded, based on information "from numerous sources" that the plaster specified by the architect, a certain "Adamant" plaster had actually been abandoned for use on the Pacific Coast, and references in San Francisco testified to its "absolute failure." The solution, quickly decided on, was to remove the ceiling plaster and replace it with square steel tiles. This proved to be an aesthetic and structural success.[14] Despite some delays in construction due to late delivery of materials (the contractor was blamed for being slow to pay the suppliers), hospital construction was very nearly complete in January 1900; only the installation of a two-story elevator, a skylight and "finish work" by painters, metalworkers, stonemasons and electricians remained. The Yard Commandant telegraphed the bureau on April 3, "Hospital building accepted and turned over to the officer in charge."[15] When all was said and done, expenditures for hospital construction equaled exactly $100,000.

The Surgeon General, in his October 4, 1900, report to the Secretary of the Navy summarized the features of the new structure:

> The circumstances under which the hospital completed in 1870 was destroyed on March 30, 1898, have been fully referred to in previous reports. The contract for the present building was awarded without delay after the preparation of plans and specifications for a thoroughly modern

Five. Early 20th Century

hospital, and the work having been completed the building was accepted on April 3, 1900, and immediately placed in order for the reception of patients. The part of the marine barracks that had been utilized for the sick was relinquished after a useful occupation of some months, and all patients transferred to the new hospital which consists of a central structure and two wings all entering their full length into the formation of the front. The wings are pavilions, each about 71 feet long and 28 feet deep containing the wards, and having transverse projections at each end in which are nurses' rooms, bath rooms, and water closets. The nurses' rooms are at the end of the wards next to the central structure and are well arranged. The pavilions[16] have two stories and a basement, and the central structure, the administration portion chiefly, has an additional story with attic. This central structure occupies about 88 feet of the front and has a depth of about 64 feet. This does not include its further extension in an addition of equal height and having an area of 37 by 60 feet. In this addition are, in the

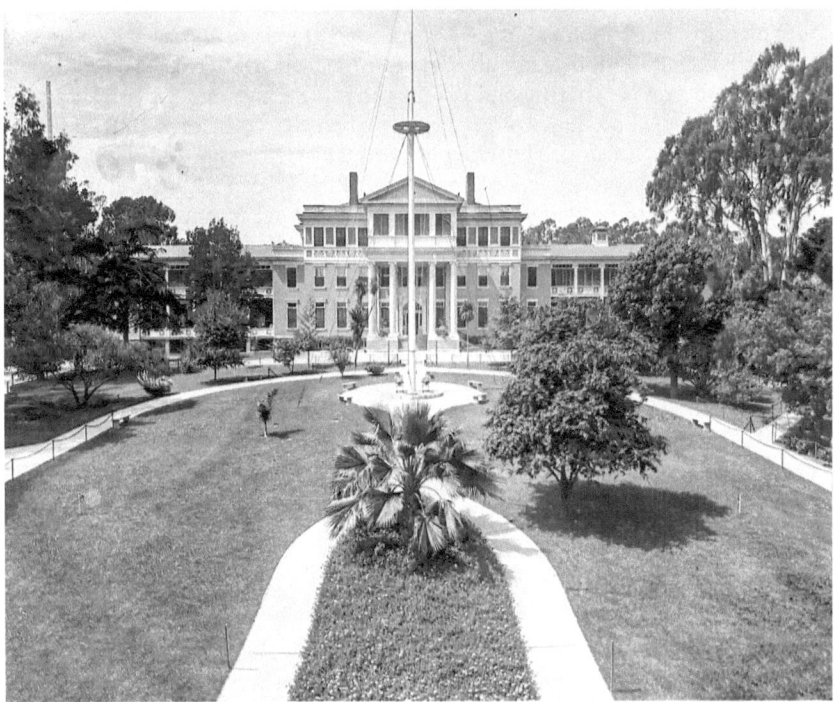

"H-1," replacement of the earthquake-damaged Naval Hospital, Mare Island Naval Ship Yard. Photo date uncertain. Mare Island Historic Park Foundation, Vallejo, California.

Part I—The Early Years

basement, storerooms, smoking room, water-closet, and space for kitchen fuel; on the first floor, general mess hall, kitchen, pantry and attendants' mess room; on the second floor, chapel, dispensary, bacteriological room, etherizing room, operating room, and recovery room; and on the third floor, eight bed-rooms with all conveniences. In the main or central portion are the administration offices, quarters for resident medical officers, and for sick officers, reception rooms, officers' mess room, library and reading room. The wards are well supplied with windows on each side, those on the front of the building opening on broad piazzas. They will accommodate 20 beds each but in an emergency the numbers can be greatly increased.

The building is of wood frame construction of the most substantial character. All the framing lumber is of Oregon or Puget Sound pine, and the finishing lumber on the interior and exterior is of California redwood. The basement story is built of brick, stuccoed and rough-cast with Portland cement, sand, and gravel. The entire building is heated by low-pressure steam from boilers outside the building. Two 42-inch Blackman fans are placed in the basement of each wing. These fans are operated by direct-connected motors of one-horse-power each and are connected with galvanized iron ventilating pipes ending in registers under each bed. The discharge ducts and flues are 25 per cent larger than the down-draft flues entering them. The entire building is lighted by electricity, and the passenger elevator is also electric, designed to lift a net load of 1,000 pounds and to have a speed to level of second floor of 100 feet per minute. A modern and extensive system of plumbing is provided and the building is piped and fitted for gas. The water pipes, fixtures, water closets, bath tubs, wash basins, discharge pipes, and sewers are all of good quality, well arranged, and of sufficient number. The entire hospital has been carefully planned and constructed and is thoroughly modern in building and equipment.[17]

From this point on, correspondence from the hospital takes on very much a work-a-day character. In May 1900, the Surgeon General wrote, "The present Naval Appropriations Bill carries an appropriation of $10,000 for a new boiler-house, boilers and equipment for the Naval Hospital." A site was duly selected,

> as best suited for the purpose ... because it is sufficiently high to permit good draining; near to the Hospital, making steam and pipe connections short; convenient to a road for coal supply; near the old building permitting the old coal bunkers to be used; and considering the prevailing winds is to the leeward of the Hospital building minimizing smoke nuisance and danger from fire.[18]

Five. Early 20th Century

The boiler house plans received the bureau's blessing on June 26. However, civilian bids for the job were not forthcoming and so, Engineer Hollyday wrote, the work could be accomplished by the yard force, with work to start "immediately." It was completed in mid–May 1901.

As with any new construction, problems inevitably arose after the craftsmen had left the scene. So it was that in late November 1900, the new hospital commander, J.A. Hawke, wrote the bureau to complain that the electric lights, especially on the second and third floors, were so dim—despite the use of 32 candle-power[19] bulbs—as to be unsuitable for reading or writing until after 9:00 p.m., when the ward lights were turned off. This was of more significance than mere convenience but one with medical implications: "In the event of a serious surgical operation at night, it is doubtful that sufficient light could be obtained to permit its being properly performed"—a clearly unsatisfactory situation. Within days, yard personnel, by a series of careful electrical measurements, isolated the problem to the segment of wiring between the switchboard and the distributing boxes being too small and not conforming with the architect's specification. A fix was instituted and the lighting problem resolved with the installation of 320 feet of wire at a total cost of $74.[20]

The hospital flagstaff was the subject of correspondence in July. Surgeon Bradley wrote the bureau to request funding to replace a flagstaff condemned by survey and removed. The unsatisfactory interim measure consisted of "a small flag ... hoisted on a boat-mast on top of the hospital." It took the bureau but ten days to request the Bureau of Construction and Repair to furnish and erect a 70-foot flagstaff with a 40-foot topmast in the hospital grounds at a cost of $922.58.[21]

An Enlisted "Hospital Corps"

By the latter part of the 19th century, many in the naval medical establishment began to see the need for well-trained enlisted medical

Part I—The Early Years

personnel. Foreign navies had already established the employment of trained medical sailors, and in 1897, the U.S. Army joined the trend. Navy Surgeon General J.R. Tryon went on record in his 1893 annual report to the Secretary of the Navy in calling for the establishment of an enlisted hospital corps to replace the method of on-the-job training for junior personnel. Surgeon General Van Reypen, in his annual report to the Secretary of the Navy of October 1, 1898, made mention, first, of the establishment—"the culmination of the efforts of the Bureau for many years"—of the Hospital Corps, stating that "it will give the service a trained corps of men who will now have some reason for remaining in the service, having a hope of promotion and advancement, as a result of faithful service, sobriety, and attention to duty." From this point forward, naval hospitals would no longer have to depend on men locally hired and trained and convalescent patients to provide care for their patients.

With the Spanish-American War imminent, Congress finally approved an act establishing a Navy Hospital Corps; it was signed into law by President William McKinley on June 17, 1898.[22] The impact of this law was first felt at Mare Island when hospital nurses Wm. A. Brame and C.D. Godfrey enlisted in the Hospital Corps and were discharged as (civilian) nurses.[23] By 1901, the Hospital Corps staff had grown to 3 Hospital Stewards, 1 Hospital Apprentice 1st Class and 16 Hospital Apprentices. Hospital Commander J.A. Hawke wrote the bureau, "I ... would request some decision from the Bureau ... in regard to the rooming and messing of ... members of the Hospital Corps." He went on to indicate that his corps staff found their sleeping quarters in a variety of ad hoc locations including the chapel for two hospital apprentices. Even the recovery room "has been turned into a sleeping space for four members of the Hospital Corps." Yard Commandant Miller forwarded this request with an endorsement indicating that "[a] pavilion for rooming of servants, Hospital Corpsmen and others is urgently needed, and the demands upon the Hospital are constantly increasing." Ever parsimonious, the bureau laconically replied,

Five. Early 20th Century

The conditions named are temporary and are due to the accumulation of members of the Hospital Corps who are intended for service in the Asiatic Station, but who are temporarily under instruction at the Hospital. The Bureau would suggest that as many members of the Hospital Corps as cannot be conveniently accommodated at the Hospital be transferred to the Receiving Ship for further instruction while awaiting transfer.[24]

I mentioned earlier that the doctors actually lived in the hospital. This naturally led to some inconveniences. For instance, early in 1901, Assistant Surgeon A.W. Dunbar wrote the bureau,

With [Hospital Commander] Dr Hawke's consent I write in behalf of Dr Orvis and myself to request permission to occasionally entertain friends in our own quarters. Dr Hawke is willing we should do so but in view of recent correspondence, he does not feel that he can give us permission to have a friend stay overnight. There is and has been no intention of using any room intended for patients in entertaining our guests.

Surgeon General Van Reypen replied, "The Bureau found it necessary to prohibit outside persons from occupying quarters in Hospital because some Medical Officers brought their relatives to live with them. This of course could not be permitted. You can say to Dr. Hawke that the Bureau has no objections to his giving permission to Medical Officers residing in the Hospital to have short visits from their friends or relatives." But he cautioned, "If these visits seem to him to be of unreasonable length, he will report the fact to the Bureau."[25]

That the new hospital was constructed entirely of fir and redwood early raised the specter of fire, and Hawke was prompted in March 1901 to write to "request that the Surgeon-General ... may be informed of the necessity for providing this hospital with an adequate number of fire-escapes. The building is entirely without such means of escape from fire at present, and in the event of fire in certain portions of the hospital, exit would be shut off—particularly in connection with the wards." He went on to request that the Navy Yard's Department of Yards and Docks (the department responsible on all Navy facilities for structural maintenance and construction of buildings, docks and other physical features) make an estimate "as to the character, number and estimated cost of same." Within

Part I—The Early Years

three weeks, Civil Engineer Hallyday submitted blueprints calling for three fire escapes at a cost of $500. The bureau quickly approved this work.[26] Subsequently, Hawke reported that the work, started in June, was completed in September 1902.[27]

Six

Toward Modernity

In mid–April 1901, Hawke received, by way of the Bureau, an inquiry from the State Department, which included a translation of a note from the "Swiss minister" asking whether the U.S. government might be amenable to meeting to revise the Geneva Convention for the Amelioration of the Condition of the Wounded in War to be convened that year. Hawke replied,

> Noted and respectfully returned to the Department ... with the recommendation that an affirmative reply be transmitted by the Navy Department.... During the recent wars questions have arisen and conditions obtained that were not contemplated at the time of the Geneva Convention. These questions and conditions necessitate additional rules for the observance of belligerents, and these rules can only be made binding by governmental assent to amendment and amplifications of the provisions of the Geneva Convention.

The convention finally did meet in 1906.[1] I do not know if the Navy had representation in Geneva, but the United States was a signatory to the final protocol, which received Senate approval in 1907.

By September 1901, Hawke was already reporting that he needed more beds. In a personal letter to Surgeon General Van Reypen on the 5th, he pointed out,

> Although built on the old foundation, the new Hospital has a less number [sic] of beds than the old—four less in each ward, by reason of a space being taken off at each end for use for a nursing room. Upon receiving patients from the [hospital ship] Solace the other day we had to send ten or fifteen out to the shack [a temporary structure that served as an administration building while the new hospital was being built] which is not a desirable place for the sick.

Part I—The Early Years

He recommended that cottages be built for the Medical Officers and pharmacist then living in the hospital "and the rooms they now occupy be utilized as wards." He added that he asked the Navy Yard civil engineer to look at the shack with a view toward making it a more suitable place to house patients. This, the engineer reported, could be done for about $2,500 but recommended that a new building be constructed instead for an additional $2,500. Hawke's own hospital carpenter thought he could renovate the building for less than $1,000. He went on, "This building should be renovated, in all events, as we have no other place for cases with contagious diseases." Van Reypen replied a couple of weeks later that he doubted that Congress would agree to spend the money for staff cottages, but he did agree to foot the bill to "fit up the shack as an overflow ward" as the hospital carpenter suggested.[2] By the end of November, Hawke was able to report that he had added four beds to each of his wards; adding the 32 beds he planned to put into the renovated shack and the eight sick officer beds, he would be able to provide care for 120 patients. "We feel that we will be able to accommodate the maximum number of patients that we are likely to have at any time in the immediate future."[3]

At the end of the year, Hawke wrote of the urgent need to retain his second assistant cook, who was to be discharged due to lack of funding. "The discharge of this man will seriously cripple our force in the kitchen," he wrote, "and if possible I would ask that the Bureau increase our monthly allowance by at least $20.00 per month. This amount itself, being a very low rate of wages for a man of any ability here." He added, "The chief cook at present employed, is an excellent man in every respect, and I should regret very much to have him leave, as he threatens to do, if he does not have two assistants." In a postscript, Hawke alluded to the fact that his cooks were Chinese: "It has been found impracticable to give the cook aid with convalescent patients, owing to racial differences." The bureau promptly telegrammed notice that the $20 monthly allowance would be made available.[4]

The shortage of beds, the need for an isolation ward and the

Six. Toward Modernity

need for houses for the junior Medical Officers came to a head early in 1902. Medical Officer of the Navy Yard, Passed Assistant Surgeon P.A. Lovering wrote to the commandant of the yard to call for a contagious ward, citing the prevalence of smallpox in the San Francisco area. Surgeon Hawke quickly expanded the discussion with this specification of details:

> The following statement is respectfully submitted for your consideration, with a view to representing the necessity for increasing the ward capacity of the Naval Hospital, Mare Island, Cal., by converting the rooms in the building, now occupied by the medical officers attached to the hospital, into wards, and for the erection in the hospital reservation, of three houses for quarters for the medical officers. The sum of $20,000 is asked for this purpose, to be appropriated by the present session of Congress.
>
> FIRST: The ward space provided for patients in the Hospital is not sufficient. There are four wards, designed to accommodate 16 beds each, or a total of 64 beds for enlisted men. One hundred enlisted men have been in this hospital at a time, during the present year, and the difficulty of finding space for 36 extra beds is easily conceived. There are, also, 8 rooms for sick officers, which, ordinarily is sufficient.
>
> SECOND: It is impossible, owing to the limited ward room to properly segregate diseases of a character requiring isolation, as tuberculosis, and it is necessary, when the hospital is crowded to its fullest capacity, to admit such patients into wards containing patients with diseases of a general character, thereby exposing them to infection. The Medical Officer in Charge has been compelled, also, to make use of the recovery-room and Chapel adjoining the operating-room to provide sleeping quarters for a portion of the members of the hospital corps, and to put two beds in rooms attached to wards for hospital corps men on duty in wards, the rooms being designed for one bed only.
>
> THIRD: This is the only Naval Hospital on the Pacific Coast, and, in consequence, patients are received not only from the Naval Station, Mare Island, Cal., U.S. Naval Training Station, San Francisco, Cal., and the vessels of the Pacific Squadron, but in addition, from the vessels of the Asiatic squadron, and the vessels and shore stations in the Philippines. As a rule a considerable number of patients are received at a time, as a result of infrequent communication, for the latter source, and the receipt of twenty or thirty patients at once, makes it a difficult problem to provide accommodations, in addition to the general average number of patients on hand. Reference is made in the Annual Report of the Surgeon General, U.S. Navy, for 1900, to the probable necessity for additional accommodations by reason of this.

Part I—The Early Years

FOURTH: The lack of ward-room makes it imperative to hold frequent surveys, recommending the discharge of men from the Naval Service for disability, many of whom would ordinarily be retained for observation and treatment for a greater length of time. During the year 1900, more cases were invalided from the service on recommendation of Boards of Medical Survey, held at the Mare Island Hospital, than at any other Hospital in the Naval Service, although at two other hospitals,—New York and Norfolk, Va.,—a greater number of patients were under treatment.

FIFTH: There has been, for some years past, a gradual increase in the number of patients received at this hospital, and especially since the Spanish-American War, and the acquisition of the Philippines,—and there is reason to suppose that, in the future, the contemplated increase of the Naval Force, will still further demand that the capacity of the hospital be made greater.

SIXTH: The medical officers attached to the hospital now occupy rooms which it is proposed to convert into wards should the erection of the quarters be authorized, thereby increasing the capacity of the building by at least 40 beds, which, with the number now available, will be adequate, at least temporarily, for such a number of patients as may reasonably be expected to be cared for in this hospital. It is estimated that $20,000 will be sufficient for the proposed alterations, and at probably less than half the cost of an annex to the present hospital, to increase the ward capacity to the same extent.

SEVENTH: The medical officers of the hospital are on duty constantly, day and night, and are therefore required to live in the hospital, or within calling distance, and the change contemplated will not only admit of increased capacity, but will also add to the health and comfort of those on whom the welfare of the patients to a great extent depends.[5]

In a personal note to the Surgeon General on February 18, Hawke noted that with 93 patients and 23 members of the Hospital Corps aboard the hospital, he was compelled to add four beds to each open ward for the extra patients and to double up the beds in the staff spaces at the ends of the wards and even to put eight beds in the chapel and the surgery recovery room to accommodate his corpsmen. He added,

> Before a great while, the [hospital ship] SOLACE will be due here again with the prospect of the receipt of a number of patients, and, in the meanwhile, no doubt, we will continue to receive patients regularly with the arrival of transports at San Francisco, besides our usual admissions from the Navy Yard and station, and from the Yokohama hospital [the U.S. naval hospital in Japan].

Six. Toward Modernity

Surgeon General Presley M. Rixey's response was to promptly request that the Secretary of the Navy add to the congressional naval appropriations money to build the infectious ward and quarters for Medical Officers—a total bill of $30,000. This appropriation received nearly unanimous support from the California delegation in the House and the Senate and passed in the Naval Act of July 1, 1902. No doubt a letter from Surgeon General Rixey to the Honorable George E. Foss, chairman of the House Committee on Naval Affairs, helped, for it laid out the need very clearly:

> In connection with the Naval Appropriation Bill under preparation in your Committee, I beg leave to again invite your kind consideration to some points of vital importance to the Bureau of Medicine and Surgery, contained in its estimates, and letters addressed to you, namely: ... increased accommodation for enlisted men in the Mare Island Hospital;—and the urgent need of a detached building at the Hospital, Mare Island, for the treatment of small pox and other cases of contagious disease.... At the Navy Yard, Mare Island, California, we have a new hospital, of modern construction, admirably adapted to its purpose, but frequently overcrowded. There are four wards, designed for 16 beds each, but the number of patients at times reaches 100, which necessitates the accommodation of 36 patients in excess of the bed space provided—a condition not conducive for securing best results. The following letter was received this morning from the Medical Officer of the Hospital: "We have in the hospital today, a total of 126 patients. Thirteen were received yesterday from the 'Wisconsin.' On the arrival of the 'Philadelphia,' I presume our number will be still further increased. Patients will be received in the meantime, no doubt, from incoming transports." I believe that no effort should be spared to have the houses built, so as to increase the capacity of the hospital. Without the detached hospital, I do not know what we would have done to accommodate the number of patients we have had, and have at present. It is absolutely imperative that the bill should go through for the proposed changes in the hospital, and the erection of the houses, and the money should be appropriated at the earliest moment. Because other quarters are not provided, the Medical Staff of the institution occupies quarters therein which could be converted into two wards for enlisted men, and I have submitted estimates for the appropriation of $20,000 to be used in converting the quarters so occupied into wards, and for the erection of suitable quarters, outside the Hospital, for the Staff. The need for increased space for enlisted men in this hospital is an existing necessity, not a prospective one, and attention has been called to it by my predecessor in his annual reports. This is the only Naval Hospital on the Pacific Coast, and receives patients from the Naval Station

Part I—The Early Years

thereon, and from the Pacific and Asiatic Squadrons. Since our occupation of the Philippines, the number of sick transferred from the Asiatic Station has largely increased. In connection with this hospital, I have also submitted an estimate of $10,000 for the purpose of providing a detached ward for the treatment of cases of small pox and other virulently contagious diseases. For such treatment the Navy has at present no facilities on the Pacific Coast, which fact of itself seems sufficient reason for the favorable action requested. The health of the personnel of the Navy is one of the most important factors of its efficiency, and the matters urged upon your Committee in this letter are believed to be essential thereto.[6]

Rixey had made it a point also to forward this same note to the Honorable Eugene Hale, a member of the Senate Committee on Naval Affairs.

Five weeks later, Washington, D.C., architect William M. Poindexter, the same man who designed the main hospital building, submitted drawings for (unspecified) changes to the second floor of the hospital, for a new contagious hospital and for two new

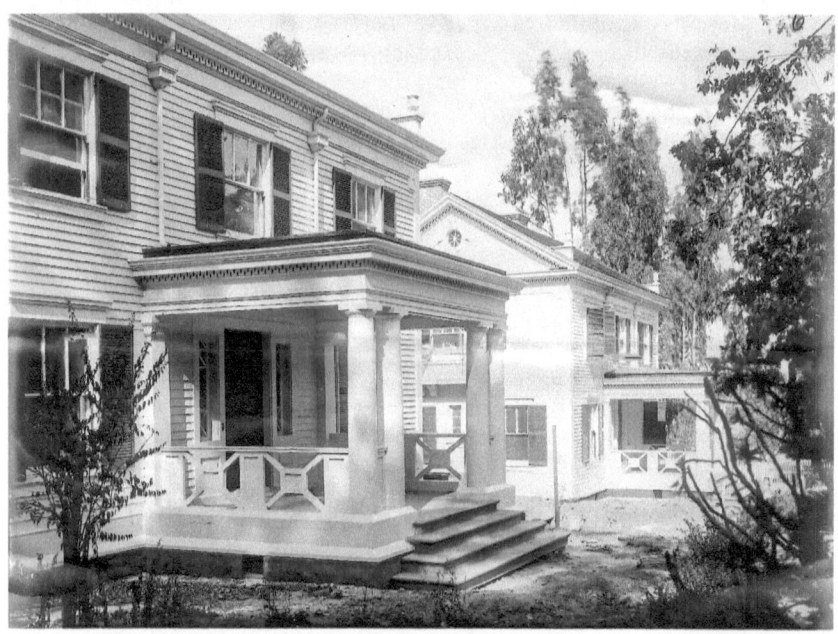

"Cottages" for Naval Hospital Executive Officer and Chief Surgeon. Official Navy photo, 1903. National Archives, Washington, D.C.

Six. Toward Modernity

officers' quarters. Preliminary bids from a Vallejo firm (Doty & Bartles) and W.N. Concannon of San Francisco confirmed the cost of around $28,000–$29,000 for the package. Duly advertised on February 3, three contractors made bids on the job, and the contract was awarded to the San Francisco firm of Hannah Brothers 17 days later. Construction commenced on March 10, 1903.[7] A year later, in an April 4, 1904, report of repairs and improvements made at the hospital, Medical Director Manly H. Simons could state that the hospital for contagious diseases had been erected, completely furnished and was ready for occupancy and that both Medical Officers' cottages had recently been occupied. He also mentioned that a bridge had been thrown up over the deep ravine separating the main hospital from the contagious disease facility.[8]

In a report of repairs and improvements for fiscal year ending June 30, 1902, Hawke mentioned that a temporary building be constructed as a furniture storage house while the main hospital was under construction for conversion to an isolation hospital of two wards, one with 20 beds (for syphilitics) and the other of 10 (for tuberculars). The building was fitted out with electric lighting, hot and cold water, steam heat and the necessary toilet and bathing facilities. Even at that, he reported, "it has been necessary to resort to the use of tents for tubercular cases."[9] Progress was slow, however, and in April 1903, the new hospital commander, Medical Director Simons, wrote the Surgeon General requesting permission to requisition three "pavilions [as isolation wards]." He penned,

> We are liable at any time to have an epidemic of mumps, measles, and diphtheria from the training station, and have no place to put more than six diphtheria, six mumps, six measles, and four small-pox cases. We still have one small-pox case in the small building used as a contagious ward. The mumps and measles are in the chapel and the convalescent ward, which are in the main building. The new building for contagious diseases will not be finished before next fall sometime, and will accommodate twelve ward and three room patients so we shall still have need for the pavilions.

He had in mind "Ducker" portable buildings, prefabricated affairs with room for 8 or 12 beds. The Surgeon General, ever parsimonious, after checking the cost and availability of the pavilions for

Part I—The Early Years

delivery to California wrote back, "Ducker houses cost twenty eight hundred dollars and cannot be procured nearer than New York. Bureau prefers Army hospital tents. Can be procured from quartermaster, San Francisco."[10] Further parsimony appeared when the Bureau disapproved Simons' request for a bicycle for use by the hospital's mail orderly to facilitate his three time daily three-mile round trip visits to the post office in Vallejo![11]

Water was on the agenda when Hospital Commander Simons wrote the Surgeon General to note that during the California dry season, he was unable to keep his water supply tank full. He anticipated additional draw on this water supply when the officers' cottages and the infectious hospital opened. He added, prophetically, "The Vallejo [Water] Company promises to run in a larger pipe so as to increase the supply to the yard and the city, but as both places are growing, this will be only a temporary expedient. The Government will have to acquire land and water-rights and have its own system eventually."[12] The Vallejo Water Company did indeed install larger pipes to supply water to the yard and the hospital, and this appears to have met the hospital's requirements—at least for a time.

In a nod to the growing acceptance of the bacterial theory of infectious disease and to protect patients in the regular hospital from contagion, a separate "Contagious Hospital" was constructed in 1903. In practical terms, it appears that the majority of the hospital's inmates were tuberculars and syphilitics; smallpox represented a small but feared portion of hospital clientele. Isolating the former here makes sense because tuberculosis is well and truly a contagious disease as the term is commonly understood, while the means of transmission of syphilis—typically by sexual contact with an infected individual—is distinctly unique and not particularly affected by the isolation provided. Perhaps there was a punitive element involved in the incarceration of the thus-miscreant sailors there. The isolation of smallpox patients would be a critical public health priority, giving time and space for the medical community to immunize the surrounding population.

Early in November 1903, Simons received a personal letter from

Six. Toward Modernity

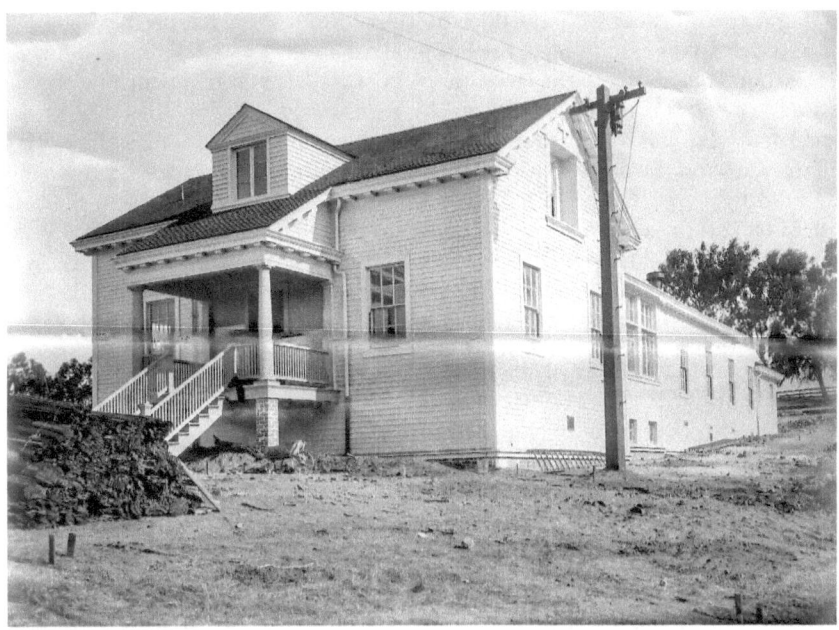

"Contagious Hospital," Mare Island Naval Hospital. Official Navy photo, 1903. National Archives, Washington, D.C.

the Surgeon General inquiring whether any cows were maintained by the hospital. He replied that, indeed, the hospital maintained two. He continued,

> It has been the custom for many years, for a butcher and ranch-owner of Vallejo, a Mr. McCudden, to let Naval Officers stationed here have cows for the pasturage; the calves are also returned to Mr. McCudden when they are five weeks old. There is quite a large herd of these cows on the Island, and new comers draw from this, or take over the cows left by their predecessors. In this way I have four, two of which are nearly dry and will soon be turned into the herd, leaving two, which is the number necessary to supply my family with milk.
>
> This custom has grown up probably from the difficulty of getting milk delivered satisfactorily from Vallejo, as there is great objection to allowing teams, which do not belong to the island, to go backwards and forwards on the ferry. My own cows have cost me more for feed than the milk would have cost. A boat is sent from the yard every week to mills nearby where Officers get grain, meal, etc., at wholesale rates.
>
> The yard has a herdsman who drives the cows backwards and forwards

Part I—The Early Years

night and morning from the open pasture. The Hospital has no such man, and the horses belonging to the Hospital, when they have the day off, and the cows belonging to the Hospital are pastured, in the field which belongs to the general Hospital enclosure. This field shows on paper, an area of 13 acres, but it is diminished in pasturage by two wooded ravines, the trees around the border and the yard and road for the contagious disease building.

   I trust that this gives the information required by your letter ... in full, my dear Doctor, though, unless you are familiar with the yard, you will not understand that the distances are great here, the Hospital is over a mile from the Yard landing, and that, in consequence, one cannot send out to replenish one's larder at short notice; therefore it is found to be almost necessary to keep cows and chickens for one's family use.

The bureau's reply was that Simons's answer was "entirely satisfactory."[13]

A poignant incident in March prompted mention of a speech given in Vallejo by President Theodore Roosevelt. Pharmacist Stephen St. John wrote to Simons to report that he had received a check from the auditor of the Navy Department for the sum of $482.43, back pay of the late Abraham Johnson, Seaman, USN, who died in the hospital. Johnson had prepared a will in which he designated the pharmacist to be the executor and further stipulated that after a proper headstone had been purchased, the remaining money should go for the purchase of athletic gear for the use of the Hospital Corpsmen on duty at the hospital. Now, this arrangement was strictly against the rules—specifically, Article 1166, Navy Regulations, 1900, which stipulated that "all persons employed in the Medical Department of the navy are prohibited ... from acting as administrator or executor for ... any patient." St. John explained that he had no foreknowledge of his having been named the executor and went on to describe that he had sought the guidance of a local lawyer, a former sailor, who had probated the will at no cost. St. John further cited a similar episode, in 1889, when Alexander White, Chief Quartermaster, USN, died, having named a medical officer as his executor, with the provision that his headstone be purchased and the remainder of his funds be used to establish a library for patients and enlisted staff at the hospital. Having demonstrated honest intent and performance

Six. Toward Modernity

of his duty regarding the deceased sailor and his will, naval authorities (the issue went all the way up to Acting Secretary of the Navy Charles H. Starling), on April 8, waived the provisions of Article 1166 in this case. It probably didn't hurt that St. John cited the Alexander White story that President Roosevelt had told a year earlier in a dedicatory speech he gave on the opening of a new YMCA in downtown Vallejo:

> I wish here to relate something told me yesterday by Secretary Moody, which shows the spirit that actuates the men of our navy. In visiting the hospital at Mare Island yesterday Secretary Moody found that there was a little library of two hundred standard novel's [sic], and a sum of money with interest amounting to $30 a year to be spent on magazines, all for the use of the patients, for the use of the enlisted men in that hospital, and he found that that was due to the action of a man now dead, who had served twenty-five years in the United States navy, had become a boatswain, and when he died had left all his small savings to be thus devoted in perpetuity to the use of his fellows who should need the hospital thereafter. His name was Alexander White, and Secretary Moody told me he intended to find out where he was buried and put a fitting stone over him if he had to pay for it himself. [Applause] That is the spirit of devotion to the flag and the country, and to one's fellows which the United States navy develops.[14,15]

In March, Simons again mentioned the need for beds in a hospital that was bursting at the seams. Citing the "increase in the Naval Force ashore and afloat and the establishment of a Training Station on this coast [at Treasure Island in the middle of San Francisco Bay]" with the attendant increase of patients from these sources and the burgeoning hospital staff, including the prospect of the need to provide accommodation for female hospital corps personnel, he suggested

> for the consideration of the Bureau that a building of two stories be put up ... and that the first story ... be arranged for members of the Hospital Corps not otherwise provided for, and the second story for a surgical ward holding 16 beds, and for a modern operating room. Also that another building be erected ... for cases of scarlatina, mumps, measles, diphtheria, and those cases of tuberculosis whose condition precluded their being put in tents.

He also pitched for two new houses, for a junior Medical Officer and for the "executive surgeon." In the same letter, he mentioned that

Part I—The Early Years

an old boiler house was in "a wretched state of repair" and recommended that it be torn down but only after buildings for a morgue, the carpenter and paint shops and a storeroom, presently housed in the old building, be constructed. The Surgeon General replied, "You are informed that it is scarcely possible that any appropriation can be secured during this session of Congress for additional buildings." He added, "The matter, however, has been noted and will receive careful consideration in the preparation of future estimates by the Bureau." He then requested requisitions and specifications for repairing and enlarging the old boiler house and for the purchase and installation of new boilers. But after a discussion of costs, Rixey took the decision to defer the project entirely "until an appropriation can be secured."[16]

The urgent need for expansion continued to occupy Medical Director Simons's attention and correspondence to the bureau, but despite two or three letters on the matter over the next several months and a formal request in his estimates for the next fiscal year for a two-story building for the corpsmen and an operating suite, a new powerhouse for two 100-horsepower boilers, a carpenter shop, a shed for services at the Naval Cemetery during the rainy season, a house for the pharmacist, a new morgue and more, Simons's pleas generated not a bit of traction back in Washington, D.C. But, in fact, Rixey in his annual report of July 1904 wrote,

> It should be remembered that the hospital establishments of the navy were designed for the accommodation of a service not exceeding the strength of 15,000, and are, consequently, in general, inadequate for the proper care of the sick and injured now numbering ... about 40,000 individuals. The necessity for hospitals of greater capacity has naturally followed. There is a need for remodeling and extending nearly all of the important naval hospitals, more particularly those at Chelsea, Mass, Newport, R.I., Norfolk, Va, and Pensacola, Fla.

Note that he made no mention of the naval hospital at Mare Island, which, as I mentioned, was bursting at the seams![17] Yet, when Simons wrote to indicate that the Vallejo Board of Trade, "very active and successful in securing work for work here on the Yard," was "anxious to request Senator Perkins, Congressmen Metcalf, Bell and others to favor anything in the way of building and improvement at

Six. Toward Modernity

this Hospital as well," Rixey offered no resistance to Simons's lobbying suggestion, adding, perhaps as a parting shot, "The Bureau has not yet decided upon recommendations for improvements made by various medical officers in charge of hospitals and no action has been taken upon the recommendation for additions, repairs, etc., made in your letter of April 20th."[18] Simons was persistent in relating the need for an expansion of the hospital, writing on the subject in May and October 1904. Finally, in July 1905, Surgeon General Rixey put the Mare Island hospital's needs into his estimates for fiscal year 1907: "For a surgical ward building for operating room and surgical cases, twelve thousand dollars; for a new building for infectious cases, eight thousand dollars; and for a new power house, five thousand dollars; in all, twenty-five thousand dollars." Then, he noted, "Since the occupation of the Philippines the number of cases treated at the Naval Hospital, Mare Island, has been so largely increased that its capacity has been constantly taxed for their accommodation."[19]

As if "in background," on July 14, the Secretary of the Navy, upon recommendation from the bureau, renewed a contract with the California State Commission in Lunacy for the care of Pacific Coast sailors (14 of them as of October) for another year.[20]

On July 18, 1905, the Asiatic Fleet Surgeon submitted an interesting report "on 58 Russian wounded, including a Prince Poutatin, and Count Iakouleff (both lieutenants), received at Cañacao[21] Hospital eight days after Russia's defeat in the Battle of Korean [Tsushima] Strait." All were received with septic[22] wounds and unreduced compound[23] fractures. Fleet Surgeon Clement Biddle wrote,

> Three Russian Cruisers have just come in after getting a disastrous beating in the Korean Straits. They slipped away, I hear, under cover of a mist, and no doubt thus saved themselves from capture in this way. To make a long story short, a lot of the wounded from these vessels have just been landed for treatment at our Cañacao Hospital.... None or almost none speaks English, the medium of communication being French, and not too good French at that. There came with these people a junior medical officer. Dr. Hiblett has given up one ward to these men and very comfortable he has made them from what I observed yesterday afternoon. Some additional baymen [corpsmen] are in attendance at Cañacao, I think, as well as P.A. Surgeon Taylor from the "Ohio." Hiblett tells me he needed baymen competent

Part I—The Early Years

to dress and bandage more than additional doctors. These patients entered the hospital about eight days after the fight, their wounds untouched from the day the first dressings were applied. All were suppurating[24] and those that I saw freely so. It quite reminded me of the condition of surgery before the advent of Listerism.[25] It was apparent that no real attempt at antisepsis by the Russian Medical Officers had been made. A rough first dressing was applied, and that's all.[26]

It's clear that this American surgeon had no respect whatever for the quality of care the Russian sailors had received.

This interesting letter appears in the hospital's correspondence file. Although directed to the Surgeon General of the Navy, it offers a glimpse into the role the naval hospital and its staff may have played in the community:

From Charles N Ellinwood, MD, President, Cooper Medical College, November 1 1905:

I beg to submit to you the purpose of Cooper Medical College to establish a department of tropical medicine here in San Francisco, and to ask your encouragement and cooperation. Our plan is to organize a school on somewhat similar lines to the London school of tropical medicine [sic], and give two courses of post-graduate instruction annually, of three months each, available to all medical men in our public and merchant services who are going to the tropics or coming in contact with tropical diseases in our seaports at home.

Great Britain has found the utility and beneficence of her school of Tropical Medicine, and we are beginning to see the necessity of cultivating by research and teaching what is being developed in the knowledge of tropical diseases among us with a view of giving the medical profession better preparation in this department of medicine and our people better protection in hygienic regulations and therapeutic measure.

We have no desire to do this for pecuniary profit and purpose [sic] to utilize our laboratories and our instructors as far as possible with the addition of such men of special training and experience as we may be able to command, and charge only such nominal fees as may be necessary for the self-maintenance of the department. Hoping that you will see some advantages in this new department in the medical teaching which may accrue to the medical officers of the navy, and also the advantages which are now apparent in this city as a permanent location for this laudable purpose, kindly give me your advice on the question and what you would be glad to do in the furtherance of our purposes.[27]

Six. Toward Modernity

No reply to this letter is found in the files. Cooper Medical School went on to become Stanford University School of Medicine. We will see the medical school and the naval hospital develop an education partnership later in this story.

Earthquake (Again—This Is California, After All)

On April 18, 1906, the San Francisco Bay Area shook for about a minute starting at 5:12 a.m. local time. Whereas the city of San Francisco was devastated, damage on Mare Island was limited. At 5:15 a.m., Assistant Surgeon F.F. Shook telegrammed the bureau, "Hospital damaged slightly by earthquake. One chimney shaken down. & some plaster knocked off of some of the walls"; a follow-up telegram corrected, "Chimneys over main building shaken down crushing in roof in three places." At 10:00 a.m., "Fitted out relief party for duty in S.F. consisting of Asst. Surgs. Shook and Jones, Shop Stewards Mosbley and Davidson, Hosp. Ap[prentice] 1c. Foss, Hospl Ap Griffin, Mc Donald and Block, with two stretchers and first aid pouches. Left hospital at 10:35." Similar relief parties were sent from the 19th through the 21st, and on the 20th, "93 beds made ready for patients from the San Francisco disaster." Forty-two patients were listed as admitted civilians. About half showed trauma or burns associated with the earthquake. The rest had a variety of ills. In a day when female nurses were not yet permitted in the Navy, five "nurses of Vallejo" did volunteer work in the hospital. The commandant of the Navy Yard directed that the Marine Band offer daily entertainment "for the benefit of the civilian refugees present in the hospital, between the hours of 3 and 4 o'clock."[28]

The Navy Yard commandant's April 18 telegram to the bureau, delayed in transmission, indicated that the hospital interior showed areas of cracked and falling plaster, and two chimneys had fallen. He didn't comment on personnel injuries.[29] The damage apparently didn't interfere with hospital operations because Navy relief parties sent to the city daily, for a week or more after the tremors, brought 45 patients back with them for care at the hospital. Not all patients

Part I—The Early Years

were suffering earthquake-related injuries. A woman civilian had surgery for appendicitis; three civilians died, none from trauma. "Repairs immediately necessary" received prompt approval on April 26, and on May 3, the Navy Department notified the yard commandant that Congress had appropriated $100,000 for the Navy Yard to include repairs to the hospital.

Hospital activities quickly returned to normal, and a May 23 letter from the hospital commander laid out some of the ongoing maintenance he had completed: "Headstones have been required for and placed in position over unmarked graves in the Naval cemetery, and the cemetery kept in good condition ... and, the hospital flag-staff was painted and wire guys overhauled and repaired."[30]

In July, the bureau sent a letter to the Medical Officer in Charge, indicating that the 1906 Naval Appropriation Act provided for "Naval Hospital, Mare Island, California: For a surgical building for operating room and surgical cases, twelve thousand dollars; for a new building for infectious diseases, eight thousand dollars; for a new power house, five thousand dollars; in all, twenty-five thousand dollars" and requesting "suggestions as to the location, size and character of the proposed buildings."[31] The new hospital commander, Medical Director R.C. Persons, replied in August proposing that a surgical building be added on to the rear wing of the main hospital and construction of three small wooden buildings, located some distance to the west of the present contagious disease building. We will see that this plan was not adopted.

On a completely different note, in March, the hospital director reported the death of the black mare "Bessie" of lockjaw, and requested permission to remove the horse's name and valuation from the hospital record. This was duly approved and "respectfully returned."[32] We will soon see that this event may have marked the beginning of a transition to internal combustion engine–driven conveyances.

The contrast of old ("Bessie" and a subsequent request for a new ambulance at $600 and a pair of horses to pull it) and new (the emerging science of medicine) is highlighted in a letter reporting

Six. Toward Modernity

"Improvements and Repairs" made to the hospital in 1907–08. An X-ray apparatus "for diagnosis, treatment and radiographic work" is at the top of the list. Importantly, however, a room previously housing hospital apprentices was converted for use as the new bacteriological laboratory, complete with "electrical wiring, and an incubator ... supplied with an automatic regulator [thermostat] devised at this hospital." A photographic outfit, perhaps for developing X-ray films, also found its way into the report, along with "a lead lined cabinet for the preservation of unused sensitive plates and paper." A headlamp for use in the eye and ear ward (instead of reflecting sunlight into ears and noses for diagnosis and treatments) modernized that area of specialty. On a more prosaic but practical note, a "two tank nickel plated dish washing machine operated by a one horse power electric motor" was installed, and it gave "entire satisfaction," for the dishes were "more safely handled and much time" was saved. Additionally, "a set of foot pedals for the Surgeon's wash bowl in the operating room has been furnished, and installed by hospital machinists." Finally, "the long distance telephone booth has been moved from the pharmacist's office to an unused door way between the Officer of the Day's Office and the main corridor, giving access to it from either side."[33]

The requisition for a "Navy Standard X-Ray Outfit," sent on October 22, 1906, was returned "approved."[34]

Concurrent with the requested X-ray unit, we are offered, from Hospital Commander Persons's report dated February 9, 1907, some insight into the treatment of tuberculosis cases in the days before antibiotics.

> All cases of pulmonary tuberculosis sent to this hospital during the year 1906 have been treated in a camp and by hygienic and sympathetic methods[35] only.
> As soon as diagnosis of the disease[36] was made after arrival at the hospital the patient was sent to the tuberculosis camp. This was located on the slope of a hill south-west from the main hospital building, where there was shelter from the prevailing west winds of the summer season. Tents were occupied during the spring of 1906, in this camp. All tuberculosis patients messed with the general mess, but at separate tables, and care was taken

Part I—The Early Years

to keep their mess-gear apart from the rest. In the late spring of 1906, the camp was removed to its present location at the hospital for infectious diseases, south of the main building. A row of six tents was placed east of this building, where some protection was obtained from prevailing winds and later, two other rows of four tents each were located on a platform farther down the slope of the hill, north-east from the building.[37]

Theodore Roosevelt, in his role as Assistant Secretary of the Navy, sent his huge statement of America as a new sea power, the Great White Fleet, on its world tour in December 1907. After port stops on both coasts of South America, the fleet's 16 battleships and auxiliaries[38] were scheduled to arrive at San Francisco in May 1908. Navy Surgeon General Rixey was anxious that Navy medicine put on its best showing. Accordingly, in February 1908, he wrote to Hospital Commander Persons to express the "desire to call your attention to the necessity of being fully prepared for the care of additional sick" and to offer extra provisions "in the way of additional medical officers, Hospital Corps men, tents, emergency repairs, etc." Within a week, Persons replied with a list of needs and closed with, "The Bureau can feel assured that the Hospital will prove equal to the work it will have to do."[39]

By the end of September, with the Great White Fleet long gone, the commanding officer could report that "our list of patients is rapidly decreasing. We have taken down and put in store the most of our tents."[40] The Navy Surgeon General's report for 1909 summarized the hospital experience: (1) greatest number of patients admitted in one day, 155 (135 of these were from the fleet's hospital ship); (2) the largest census in any one day, 265; (3) 213 major and 123 minor surgeries "of varying degrees of gravity" were performed; and just 14 deaths, despite a "broad range of disease conditions ... includ[ing] many very serious cases." The Surgeon General made particular mention of the extensive use of the hospital's laboratory, "used as an aid in diagnosis and treatment, 2,241 examinations having been made."[41]

A July report of "Improvements and Repairs" of the hospital told of the number of additional beds (400) and accoutrements the hospital had procured "to supply the needs of the additional sick from the Battle Ship fleet, making with the vessels of the Pacific fleet, approximately 25,000 men."[42]

At the end of 1908, the Surgeon General sent a circular letter to all hospital commanders to solicit reports on defects and deficiencies in a broad range of hospital facilities and services. Most interesting in Persons's reply was the comment, "An automobile ambulance will be of immense service."[43] Yet another push to the future of modern medical care on the Pacific Coast.

"Nurses (Female)" for the Navy

As I mentioned in an earlier chapter, the Navy was traditionally a male-dominant organization. Even in the hospital setting, first convalescent patients, then trained medical assistants cared for patients as they recovered from illness or from surgery. The British statistician and social reformer Florence Nightingale was influential in the development and evolution of the profession of (female) nursing by establishing nursing schools in Britain. A Nightingale-mentored woman, Linda Richards, brought the idea back to the United States and established early training programs here. By the end of the 19th century, the profession of nursing was well established in the civilian sector. The Army, having hired contract nurses to great benefit for soldiers suffering from the tropical diseases associated with service during the Spanish-American War, requested Congress to establish a Nurse Corps, legislation for which was passed in 1901. The Navy's experience with female nurses dates back to the Civil War, when four Sisters of Mercy cared for men in USS *Red Rover*. During the Spanish-American War, three female medical students from Johns Hopkins University and a premed student from MIT were contracted as Navy nurses but only for "the duration." They left with the thanks of the Surgeon General at the end of hostilities. The Navy had learned its lesson, however, and every year thereafter the Surgeon General passed his request for establishment of a Navy Nurse Corps up the chain of command for submission to Congress. Finally,

Part I—The Early Years

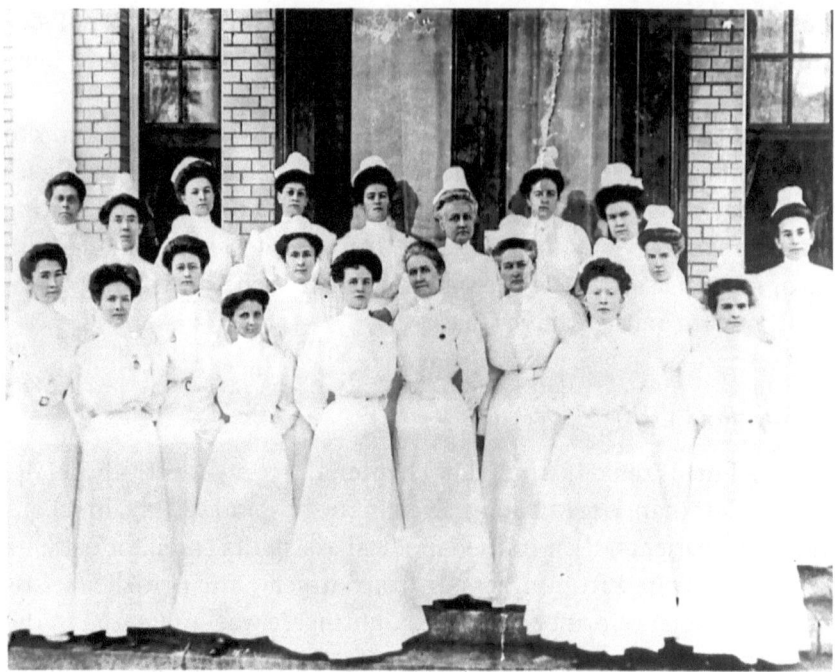

"The Sacred Twenty." Official Navy photograph of the first 20 nurses in the Navy. Martha Pringle is third from the right in the front row. Official Navy photograph, circa 1908. Downloaded from the Navy History and Heritage Command (https://www.history.navy.mil/content/history/nhhc/our-collections/photography/us-people/b/bowman-j-beatrice/nh-52960.html).

in 1908, Congress agreed. Twenty nurses were initially recruited and assigned to the naval hospital in Washington, D.C., for their Navy indoctrination.

Assistant Surgeon General N.C. Braisted wrote a personal letter to Hospital Commander Simons early in December to tell him that Miss Martha Pringle, "one of the best, if not the best of the nurses in the Corps," would be sent to Mare Island. He added, "You will find her an exceptionally fine woman." Braisted expected Miss Pringle to bring a corps of women nurses to the West Coast as soon as possible and to scout out suitable living spaces for them. Along with details of how the nurses might be housed and finances provided for this, Braisted included the encouraging message, "These woman nurses

Six. Toward Modernity

have proven to be of exceptional value in the hospitals already supplied, and the Surgeon General felt that Mare Island, at least, on the west coast should be supplied as soon as possible." Later, making one believe that Braisted anticipated some resistance, he added, "I feel sure that, as soon as you have had the assistance of these women in your serious cases and the running of the hospital, you will feel that you have a most valuable adjunct in them." Nurse Pringle's pay would be $65 a month.[44] Simons promptly replied in the most affirmative tone, reassuring that he would "arrange matters as nearly as possible to the satisfaction of the Bureau, the nurses and the hospital," though he did point out that decent housing in Vallejo might be hard to procure for the amount of money ($37.50 per month budgeted by the bureau). Two days before Christmas 1909, Simons wrote to say that Miss Pringle had arrived and was engaged in "hunting available apartments" and that she found the crossings and streets very muddy and traveling accordingly uncomfortable. He added that the nurses would have a three- or four-mile commute each way (this in horse-drawn carriages), that rental in town would cost $75 a month minimum, and that he'd asked the commandant of the Navy Yard that a house just outside the hospital compound be made available for temporary use. For a variety of bureaucratic reasons, this did not come to pass despite Miss Pringle's firm opinion.[45]

In January 1909, the Surgeon General wrote to Persons at Mare Island to indicate the bureau's intent to order six "nurses (female)" to Mare Island and inquired about the availability and adequacy of housing for the women. Persons replied that, by moving staff around, he could find suitable quarters for them in the hospital itself, but he urged the bureau "to give early consideration to the erecting of a separate building," especially if the bureau anticipated sending more than six. In February, Mare Island appeared on a list of hospitals receiving Secretary of the Navy approval for said construction.[46,47]

In a June 15, 1909, personal and handwritten note to Surgeon General Rixey, Simons penned, "The work on the new [surgical] ward is going steadily but slowly.... The workmen are slow but they do good work. Perhaps it evens out that way, but I feel a powerful inclination sometimes to get in among them and make them, in plain English, sweat a little. It would do them good and I know it would relieve me."[48] He added that dirt removed from the excavation from the new structure was used to fill in a ravine behind it. (No evidence of this ravine exists in 2023.)

In February 1910, Simons wrote to the Surgeon General,

> Sir, the recent order of Hospital Corps men to Canacao has taken from us our best operating-room man, and I trust that you will find it convenient to give for this place Miss Isabelle Baumhoff, now second only in the operating-room at the Annapolis [Naval] Hospital.... Miss Baumhoff is personally agreeable to Miss Pringle who is quite lonesome. It is a good time, now that a change has been made, to induct a nurse into this very important position without undue friction.

The bureau granted rapid approval for this move.[49] Six other nurses arrived during April and May, firmly establishing the Nurse Corps' presence on the West Coast. Later, in June, a notation appears indicating, "Navy Nurse Corps (female) West coast applicants for appt. as nurses will report with testimonials etc. to M. Isld Hospital for scrutiny and recommendations on fitness for Corps." Hand entered on this note, "Miss Anna Turner, Mare Isl. Cal first permit issued under this arrangement."[50]

Following the saying "You can never have too much of a good thing," Simons wrote the bureau in September to pitch for more nurses:

> At present we have as follows—Nurses..8, including chief nurse; number of wards inclusive of new wing..14—of these 7 do not need nurses; these are—4 venereal wards, the tents, 3 contagious wards and 1 locked ward, leaving 7 wards for the female nurses—2 surgical and 5 medical. There should be three for each, but we can do with two for each, and there should be one for each diet kitchen (2), and one for the operating room, making for 24 as the maximum and 17 as the minimum, exclusive of the chief nurse.[51]

Nurses (female) had clearly "arrived" on the West Coast, and thus began a long and distinguished record of care that lasted nearly half a century.

In February 1910, Simons wrote to the Surgeon General, "The new, or surgical wing will be ready for occupancy this summer. The work is proceeding in the usual slow but thorough manner of Navy Yard work."[52] He went on to pitch the addition of a second story on the power house. This would provide quarters for civil employees, then domiciled on the third floor of the hospital. "These hospital rooms are desired to make into quarters for sick officers, a diet kitchen, etc. There are now only eight rooms for sick officers in this hospital and there are frequently ten to twenty officers under treatment."

In a separate communication, Simons wrote to the Surgeon General, noting that the new gashouse addition "will provide rooms for 18 employees, which is the number now in the hospital, but as 8 of these employees are Chinese, it is deemed by the Medical Officer in Command to be advisable to put only the white employees in this building, and to leave the Chinese in their present rooms in the basement of the hospital."[53]

As we've observed earlier, due to a relative lack of workers, labor in California was (is) expensive. December 1910 seems to have been Medical Inspector Simons's month of high costs, as he wrote separate letters to the bureau asking for an increase in pay for his laundrymen from $25 per month to $35 for the lead man and from $20 to $30 for three others; for the machinist ("has charge of the water and steam-piping, electric wiring, machinery and metal work in general") a $10 raise, noting that machinists earn "from $83 up" in the local economy.[54]

One cost of America's early colonialism is expressed in the Surgeon General's annual report of 1911:

> The increased personnel of the Navy and the proximity of the Naval Hospital at Mare Island, Cal., to San Francisco, which is the port of entry of most of those who are invalided from our insular possessions and from the Asiatic Station, cause this hospital to be second in importance only to that at Norfolk. Despite the recent completion of the new wing at the institution, the medical officer in command states that "the hospital accommodations are insufficient for the rapidly growing needs of the hospital. A new ward, increase in size of the sick officers' quarters, a nurses' home, and quarters for civil employees, some of whom must at all times be at the hospital, are urgently needed at this station."[55]

Part I—The Early Years

Food was on the mind of P.A. Lovering, the new hospital commander, when he wrote in July 2011 that his four cooks had to provide for over 300 patients and staff. This work was made more difficult because the messrooms had seating for only 120, requiring a second seating at each meal. The bureau promptly approved two additional men at $35 a month.[56] In another nod to modernity, Lovering requested approval of a vacuum cleaner ($130 added in pencil) and tools: "In submitting this requisition, I would say that I believe the cleaner necessary to keep rugs and fittings of the sick Officers' quarters and hospital generally, free from dust. In an institution of this size, a vacuum cleaner is considered indispensable." The bureau replied recommending, "the Santo Vacuum Cleaner," indicating that this device had been in use five days a week for a year at the New York naval hospital with "no repairs whatever." And the best part, it could be had for $112.50, "delivered at the Naval Hospital, Mare Island."[57]

In January 1912, the Secretary of the Navy promulgated "General Order 148," labeled "Liability Act," with this short description: "Removal of civilian sick by Government conveyance or necessary admission to Naval Hospital at 50cts per diem, favor of Naval Hospital Fund."[58] It had long been a custom that civilian workers could be admitted if on-the-job injury required emergency care.[59] But correspondence after issuance of the general order took a different tack—that regarding the admission of female civilians and males for non-urgent care. Hospital Commander Gates wrote in June 1913, commenting that "the fact of civilians having been so admitted is widely discussed and there are indications that the number of applicants will considerably increase." He went on, "The civilians admitted since I have been here have all requested it for their own convenience and none was an emergency case.... Male civilians have been cared for in wards and have not always been appreciative of their privileges. One hernia case [note, an "elective" surgery in most cases] was highly indignant when, ten days after operation, was placed on house diet and his special beefsteaks, etc., stopped." Surgeon General Stokes replied, "Each case places a burden upon the hospital in many other ways which it not be prepared to bear without

Six. Toward Modernity

detriment to the service's interests. I count upon you, therefor [sic], to cooperate with the Bureau in deprecating, as tactfully as may be, the continuance of this practice except, of course, under [in cases of grave emergency where no other facilities are at hand]."[60]

The bulk of correspondence from this point until 1916 was around the desperate need for more bed space, especially for patients suffering from contagious diseases. Typical is this letter from M.F. Gates to Surgeon General Braisted in February 1914:

> In my annual report I noted that the pressing need of this institution at present is an increase of capacity. For some years hospital tents have been used and although they are at times very uncomfortable we have been obliged to keep a number, averaging about ten, occupied so far during this very rainy winter.... If you could put a rider on the Naval appropriations bill to authorize the expenditure of $15,000.00 or $20,000.00 from the Naval Hospital Fund for the construction of isolation pavilions, in view of the imminent increase in the number of Marines at this station and the probability of the fleet visiting this coast, the expenditure to be under your direction, we will do our part.... Some provision must be made soon as we are caring for from 190 to 210 patients most of the time now and have increased our ward capacity by putting in folding cots in addition to the normal number of beds. If we could get fifty or a hundred more patients, we will have to occupy the corridors and basement which would not be at all satisfactory.[61]

The bureau ultimately relented despite budgetary restrictions, agreeing to the construction of five "temporary" pavilions, which Gates reported as "in progress" in January 1915.[62] The Mare Island Naval Hospital section of the Surgeon General's annual report to the Secretary of the Navy for fiscal year 1916, ending June 30 of that year, noted, "The five new pavilion wards for permanent use as well as to provide for the expected arrival of the Atlantic Fleet have been completed and are in use."

In an interesting example of innovation at Mare Island, the surgeon in command observed, "The commissary department has been experimenting with the cafeteria system of messing convalescent patients and hospital corpsmen. The results achieved have seemed to justify the claims made for it by various officers, both from convenience and economy."[63]

Part II

The 20th Century
Responding to World Events

Seven

First "Test of War"

"Since April 6 the Navy of the United States has been undergoing the test of war."[1] So opens Navy Secretary Josephus Daniels's annual report for fiscal year 1917. But it appears that the Mare Island Naval Hospital wasn't much tested, as correspondence from the hospital commander consists almost exclusively of the proposed construction of two-story ward buildings, the result of generous congressional "emergency hospital" appropriations. In general, naval expenditures rose amazingly, from $8 million a month in 1916 to about $60 million in 1917. With that came a proportional increase in the number of naval personnel, from about 73,000 officers and men before the war to nearly 270,000 by the end of fiscal year 1917.[2] Daniels specifically commended the work of Navy doctors, nurses and hospital apprentices in responding to the large increase of men coming into the Navy: "The unprecedented cold spring made for increased cases for treatment, and contagious diseases brought in by new recruits, the necessity for new quarters, and the provision of good sanitary conditions called for self-sacrifice and increasing effort by the medical staff."

As part of the huge expansion of spending for the Navy listed above, provision was made for construction of "emergency hospitals," not in the sense we think of them as places for emergency medical care but rather as construction responding to the "emergency" demands of wartime "at a cost of $4,000,000."[3] Mare Island benefited from this program, too, with the construction of four two-story pavilions.[4] While the Mare Island hospital didn't see a significant number of war casualties—the war being a European affair with

Part II—The 20th Century

large impact on East Coast medical facilities—the construction was not for naught as we will shortly see.

But the war had an impact on Vallejo. The population roughly doubled, from around 11,000 in 1910 to around 21,000 in 1920.[5] This increase can be attributed largely to the increase in naval shipyard workers and their families, attracted by increased shipbuilding activity. In addition, the Marine Corps operated its only boot camp west of the Mississippi at Mare Island from 1917 until 1923. In response, downtown Vallejo, which abuts the Napa River on the other side of which is the Navy Yard, developed a lively enterprise catering to the needs and desires of Marines and sailors—some of which were not in their best interest. Despite Navy Secretary Daniels's appeal to the governor of California, "there lies upon us jointly the duty of protecting these young men from that contamination of their bodies which will impair their efficiency in service, blast their lives for the future, and return them to their homes a source of danger to their communities."[6] Vallejo authorities' efforts to control the trade in alcohol, gambling and prostitution didn't rise to high standards, so we can be assured that at least some of the "contagious wards" at the hospital were occupied by men who indulged in the local resources. Hospital Commander T.A. Berryhill alluded to problem in a September 17, 1917, letter to the Surgeon General:

> There are at all times under treatment at this hospital several hundred convalescent patients, also a great number of hospital corpsmen and enlisted men of the Reserve.... I request that a recreation hall of about five thousand square feet ... be authorized in connection with the emergency construction about to begin. This is needed as an aid to discipline, and to promote the contentment, welfare and happiness of the enlisted personnel.... The advisability of keeping all patients on the hospital reservation is obvious, and the absolute lack of any provision for amusement or recreation renders this difficult at the present time.

Surprisingly, the Bureau of Yards and Docks[7] demurred, replying, "On account of the lack of funds, it was decided to do nothing at present about a recreation hall."[8] (Handwritten below this message was, "If funds be available, we can build the recreation structure later.") The new hospital commander, Ammen Farenholt, struck

Seven. First "Test of War"

on a typically "military" solution in March 1919, with the institution of a Marine guard to provide sentries at the hospital gates and a patrol for the hospital reservation. Farenholt shortly later observed, "The marine guard ... is performing very valuable service—especially in preventing unauthorized persons from entering the grounds and detecting improper attempts to leave the compound by patients, hospital corpsmen and civil employees." He added, "There is also an added air of smartness and efficiency and greater security to the buildings."[9]

Wartime emergency appropriations bought several desperately needed facilities to the hospital complex, variously reported in Farenholt's weekly, semi-official letters: a mortuary (completed in February 1918), corpsmen quarters (February) and nurses' quarters (April). Farenholt also converted a condemned Hospital Corps quarters into a recreation hall, library, canteen and theater (May). He commented on the latter, "Much interest is being shown by the personnel here in its completion and, as absolutely nothing of the kind now exists here, its completion will fill a long felt want and secure a degree of contentment not known before."[10] In July, he reported the inaugural performance (libretto and music written by Assistant Surgeon E.G. Dickinson) in the theater, with a cast of corpsmen, attended by most of the officers of the Navy Yard and many from San Francisco, and in August, the first "clinical" (by which I assume he meant "medical educational") moving pictures attended by "a large and appreciative audience."

The Influenza Pandemic—True Test of the War

We now know that the 1918–1919 influenza pandemic was the worst public health disaster of the 20th century. American deaths from the flu were an estimated 675,000, by far more than deaths from all our wars in that century.[11] The infection was not typical of usual influenza in that it affected young adults of military age with particular virulence. There are frequent descriptions of young soldiers or sailors presenting to morning sick call feeling poorly, then turning blue and dying of an overwhelming lung inflammation by four in the afternoon. The cause of this disease was a mystery to the doctors of the time. It was surely contagious, but the causative factor could not be identified. Viruses were only identified in the 1930s, well after the pandemic had cleared. We now know that this was, in the majority of cases, an inflammation of the lungs, not an infection per se. The inflammation was due to an immune overreaction to the virus, referred to as a "cytokine storm."[12] Navy Surgeon General Braisted identified the entry point of the flu among Navy personnel to be the Commonwealth Pier in Boston, when, on August 27, 1918, three cases of influenza were entered to the sick list. From the East Coast, the infection spread centrifugally across the nation, arriving in Chicago on September 16. A week later, the doctors at Mare Island received a dispatch from the Great Lakes Naval Training Center in which the Chicago Medical Officers described their experience: 20 percent of the installation's manpower complement would become infected, and of those afflicted, 10 percent would develop "pneumonia."[13] A week later, Farenholt wrote in his semi-official letter of September 26 that "preparations have been made for the expected appearance of the epidemic of influenza; all available tentage is being set up, extra cots purchased and plans adopted to meet this emergency.... No case has appeared at this date."[14] A week later, just 12 cases had appeared for treatment. Farenholt wrote that a smallpox outbreak had occurred in the nearby city of Vallejo and that three of these were Navy Yard civilian workers. California State health authorities had put the "Vallejo Central Hospital" (actually, the home of local physician John J. Hogan) in quarantine, thereby making it unavailable for the care of "the general public" in the city. He hoped "that no transfers of medical officers, nurses and hospital corpsmen will be made ... as in the presence of an epidemic we cannot afford to decrease our complement. There are 746 patients cared for here now" (most of these were not flu cases).[15] Two weeks later, the doctors, nurses and corpsmen were caring for 500 cases of influenza and 100 cases of "pneumonia." On October 25, Farenholt wrote that the

Seven. First "Test of War"

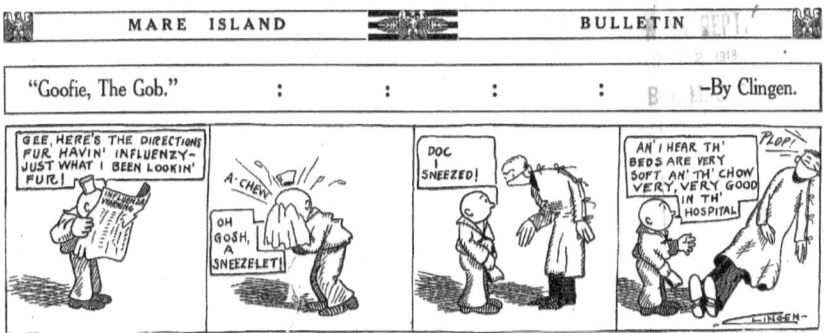

Influenza Cartoon, "Goofie, the Gob—by Clingen." Published in the *Mare Island Bulletin*, October 1918. National Archives, Washington, D.C.

hospital had experienced 840 admissions, 115 cases of pneumonia and 68 deaths, including one doctor, Lt R.C. Christiansen, chief of Laboratory Service ("more especially felt"). On a lighter note, "as an indication of the popular impression of the food and comfort supplied by the hospital," Farenholt enclosed a cartoon clipping from the *Mare Island Bulletin*.

In the meanwhile, the flu hit the city of Vallejo very hard. As I noted earlier, the city's population had doubled as a result of wartime activity, so housing was extremely tight. In fact, many boarding houses were "hot-bunking"—that is, sleeping two or three men in shifts in the same bunk—Navy Yard workers. In addition, authorities were slow in closing down theaters and dance halls, and war bond drives encouraged large groups of people to congregate. The local medical community was overwhelmed, with individual doctors taking 30 calls a day or more to make house visits. Entire families were afflicted with the flu, and death was a frequent visitor. The local civilian hospital, Dr. Hogan's home, was fully occupied by smallpox patients—there was an epidemic going around town—and Navy doctors were sent out to help in the vaccination effort to control its spread. The local Catholic bishop offered his school, closed because of the epidemic, as a hospital. The naval hospital dispatched doctors and corpsmen to care for patients—men, women and children—there. In the end, more than 250 people received care at "St. Vincent's Naval Hospital."[16]

Part II—The 20th Century

The cause of the flu was a mystery to the medical men. Viruses had not yet been described (with the exception of the tobacco mosaic virus, a huge one of its kind). Previous flu-like epidemics had been attributed to bacterial infections due to a bacteria then called *Haemophilus influenzae*. Accordingly, much treatment was aimed at attacking or preventing this infection. Antibiotics were still 30 or more years in the future, so the best remedies the doctors had were such things as spraying carbolic acid (phenol) in sailors' throats.

The epidemic clearly started to wane toward the middle of November. It helped that the Marine Corps were not sending any new recruits to the training center on Mare Island, and by the end of the month influenza admissions were down to about four a day and total flu cases in hospital were about 94. In mid–December, Farenholt wrote, "Influenza is annoying and this first recrudescence does not show signs of lessening. We have today 167 cases. Their severity is markedly less than that of a month ago." A week later,

> Influenza admissions have steadily risen, and we have now two hundred (200) cases. The virulence, however, … is very markedly less than that noticed in the initial wave. There are about twenty (20) cases of pneumonia, and there have been no deaths since 24 November at this hospital from that cause. In fact, the present cases have little similarity clinically to the former ones.[17]

By December 28, things had become decidedly more relaxed. Farenholt wrote, "Besides the ordinary routine work of the hospital, the chief interest this week was centered in a friendly rivalry of officers, nurses, and hospital corpsmen, in hospital decorations. The Amusement Fund obtained a silver cup, to be competed for by the twenty-two wards." The winning ward got to hold the cup in a glass display case until the competition in the next year. Farenholt added that his staff had made several truck trips into "surrounding counties" to obtain trees, greens, mistletoe, and so forth, all funded by the Amusement Fund.

Two more flu-related deaths among hospital staff received notice: on January 4, 1919, of Miss Drusilla Caterline, nurse, of pneumococcal septicemia[18]—she was buried at the Mare Island Naval

Seven. First "Test of War"

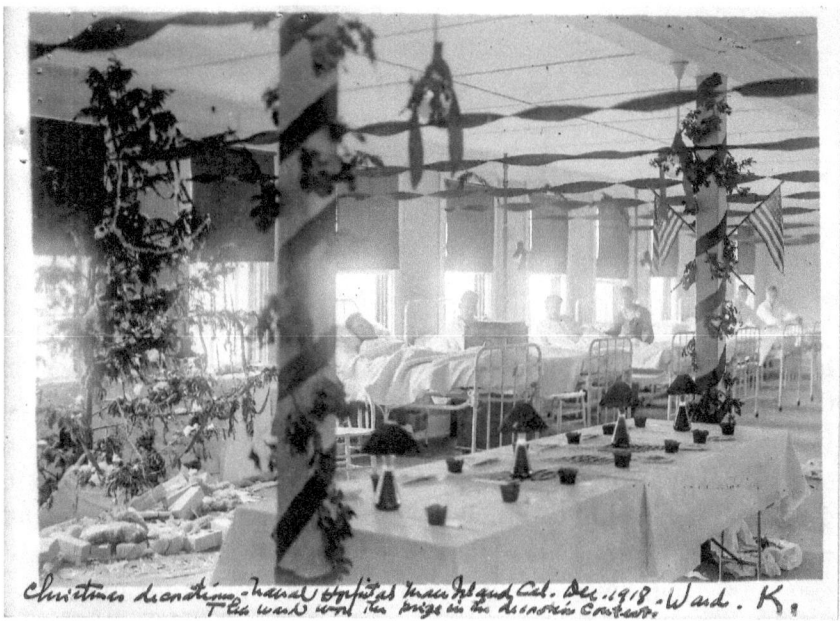

"Christmas Decoration—Naval Hospital, Mare Island, California, 1918. Ward K. This ward won the prize in the decoration contest." Photo by Hospital Commander Captain Ammen Farenholt. National Archives, Washington, D.C.

Cemetery[19] with full naval honors, and on January 10, of Lieutenant (J.G.) Henry V. Bogue, Medical Corps—"He was our specialist in eye, ear, nose and throat disease. He had been recently enrolled from Los Angeles and was not only an excellent specialist, but a general favorite of all."[20]

Eight

Interbellum

The flu manifested a mild resurgence in January 1919. Hospital Commander Farenholt, in his weekly semi-official letters back to the bureau early in the month, noted the prevalence, with 141 cases in hospital on the 10th. Once again, the Catholic school served as a civilian hospital for just a couple of weeks, and the yard commandant directed the hospital to supply, "temporarily," the services of eight nurses and one ambulance. Everyone was relieved when the contagion waned with the approach of spring, and hospital life settled into a quieter routine.

In the same letter, Farenholt returned to a common Mare Island theme: the need for more and better facilities. In this case, he referred to reporting in "various newspapers" that the Pacific Fleet might be reestablished "in force," with the number of personnel meeting "practical war strength, vastly greater than that of pre-war days."[1] Manpower became a concern of the hospital commander, too. The end of the war in Europe resulted in a rapid demobilization of nearly 2 million men. Of course, they had to be transported back to the United States in ships, and it fell to the Navy, as Surgeon General Braisted put it, to pay "strict attention to its main concern—the health of the Navy and of the several million men of the Army committed to the care of the Navy while in peril on the deep."[2] This meant the transfer of large numbers of enlisted Hospital Corpsmen to serve in the transport ships bringing the troops back home. Moreover, doctors, nurses and enlisted men, "who promptly left their work to join the colors and play their part in the furtherance of the country's cause," were now eager to return to their civilian occupations.

Eight. Interbellum

As early as January 24, 1919, Hospital Commander Farenholt complained that "repeated orders to transfer all available enlisted force for sea service, chiefly for transfer to the East coast for transport duty and also the requirements of disenrollment orders, have caused us to lose men previously considered almost indispensable."[3] He continued to complain about personnel losses—now also including doctors and nurses—for the rest of the year. And he worried frequently about an expected influx of patients when the now greatly enlarged Pacific Fleet pulled into the Bay Area in August. In fact, the patient census more than doubled, from 403 in February to an average of 853 in December 1919.[4]

Over the summer, a new postwar national program appeared on the scene with real impact on hospital operations. The first indication, in July, was receipt of notice from the bureau "to be prepared to accommodate up to 200 War Risk Insurance patients."[5] As a result of this additional patient load, Farenholt wrote, "[We] anticipate a very active and possibly strenuous future."

There was good news, too. Thanks to a generous stream of funding during the war, Farenholt could report the opening, in August, of a new building built specifically as a laboratory facility. This facility reflected at once an increase in the application of "science"—chemistry, bacteriology and hematology—to the practice of medicine and the increasing numbers of laboratory examinations the doctors were ordering. Farenholt's letter of September 1919 is instructive: "Laboratory Examinations have been as follows: July—2185; August—2469; September—3455." (That's more than 100 a day, and this in the day before automation.)[6]

One of the themes of this history is the notion of Medical Officers wearing two "hats": one of Navy officer, whose interest is in benefiting the Navy, and one of physician and surgeon, whose interest is the welfare of his patients. I think Ammen Farenholt shows how the "doctor hat" won out. Not only did he vigorously advocate for adequate staffing of his hospital in a time of postwar budget cuts and reductions in force, but he arranged for a variety of social and recreational events and entertainments. In addition, he saw to adding such

Part II—The 20th Century

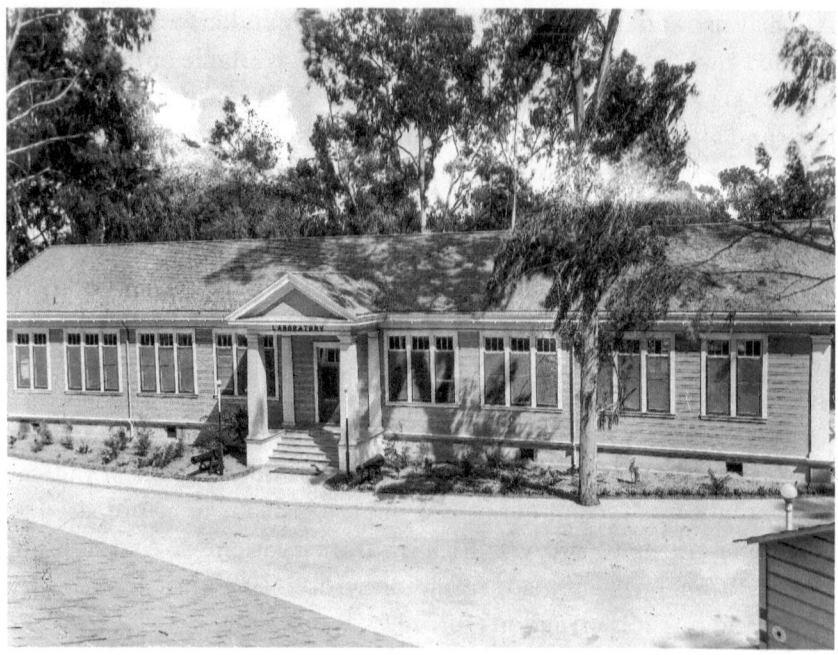

Laboratory building, Mare Island Naval Hospital, circa 1919. National Archives, San Bruno, California.

features in the hospital landscape as lighted fountains to enhance the healing environment. In February, Farenholt was happy to learn that the Surgeon General had approved construction of a Red Cross recreational facility, "a pet project" of his. The work was rapidly accomplished, and the building, which housed a post office, officially opened in October 1919. Sadly, this lovely facility was destroyed by fire in October 1927, only eight years after it opened. It was never replaced.

Farenholt's attention even fell to the level of correspondence about ambulances. Typically, in 1919, he complained about the loss of vehicles to accident (a Studebaker) or transfer to other naval hospitals (a Cadillac). He also wrote an appreciation for another Cadillac ambulance sent to Mare Island.

Another theme of this history is "Innovation on Mare Island." A nice example of this appeared in correspondence, in April 1920, from

Eight. Interbellum

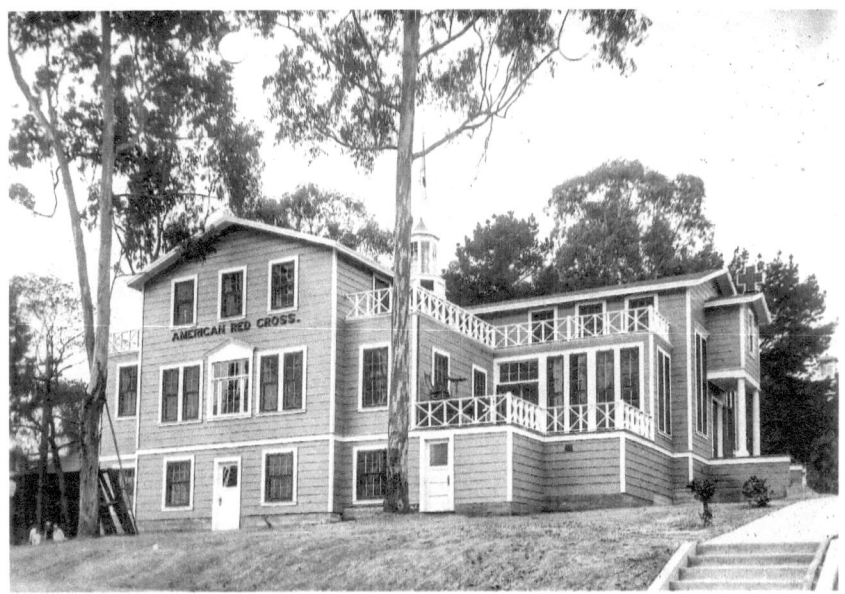

Red Cross building, Mare Island Naval Hospital, circa 1920. The sailors' post office was located in this building. National Archives, Washington, D.C.

Surgeon General Braisted to the chief of naval operations regarding a request for a motorboat ambulance from the receiving ship in Boston that could make the run from Hingham to the naval hospital in Chelsea. Accompanying his endorsement of this request and a recommendation that similar boats be provided to naval stations in Puget Sound, Washington, and San Diego, California, he wrote,

> The ambulance boat in use at Mare Island has given satisfactory service. This ambulance boat was constructed at the Mare Island Navy Yard by altering the design of the 65-foot motor launch to accommodate patients in stretchers. It is recommended that if the Navy Department approves the allowance and assignment of ambulance boats to the above mentioned stations, that the same type of motor ambulance as now used at Mare Island be approved.[7]

The record shows that Mare Island workers produced two more ambulance boats, both of which saw service in Norfolk, Virginia. Mare Island's boat served in the San Francisco Bay until 1939.

Part II—The 20th Century

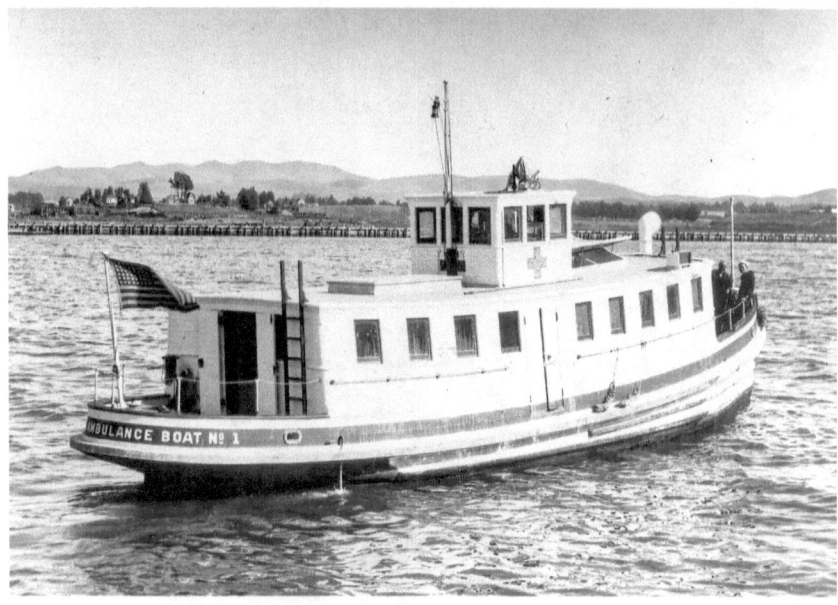

Ambulance boat #1 (VH-1), circa 1920. An example of innovation at Mare Island Naval Ship Yard. National Archives, Washington, D.C.

I've observed earlier that the labor situation on the West Coast was, from the beginning, a difficult one of shortage and high wages. One way hospital commanders dealt with this was by hiring immigrant labor, in particular Chinese and later Filipino workers. Farenholt nicely captured the situation in his May 31, 1920, semi-official letter to the bureau:

> The Bureau's letter … concerning reduction, owing to limited funds, comes to us at a most unfortunate time as our civilian employees are with the greatest difficulty held here at their present rates of pay. The labor market on this Coast is very unsettled, and the Chinese especially are able to command considerably higher wages than we are able to give them. For these reasons labor is "floating," discontented and our vacancies cannot be filled.[8]

Earlier, Farenholt had reported, "Educational classes for our Chinese employees are being started. This is partly necessary to make this class of employees contented and to keep them from leaving us for the higher wages being paid outside."[9]

I've remarked before that the hospital commanders, almost from

Eight. Interbellum

the opening of the main hospital building ("H-1"), worried about the risk of fire in wooden structures. In a letter requesting the service of additional carpenters for maintenance work, Farenholt remarked that the hospital reservation had 45 separate (wooden) buildings with "over 2600 windows and 257 doors." In June 1919, he wrote,

> The question of fire protection of this hospital and its 45 wooden buildings is a most important one and one which causes us all the greatest anxiety and apprehension. All wiring, chimneys, etc. have been checked up by yard experts and the fire chief has inspected us several times and has nothing to suggest except our fundamental error of construction. Still those buildings, and most especially the three story main hospital building, are a dangerous fire risk.[10]

Among the recommendations in an inspection report by Admiral A.M.D. McCormick in July was to "replace main hospital and all wooden buildings that may be desirable for retention, by fireproof structures."[11] In April 1924, Inspector Rear Admiral George H. Barber wrote that he "emphasizes the fire hazard constituted by the many wood frame buildings in the complex." A short-term and absolutely necessary approach to the problem was the construction of fire escapes enclosed in concrete shafts. The constant worry about fire rose to the level of the Surgeon General's attention when the new Surgeon General Edward Stitt, in a July 1922 letter to the Bureau of Yards and Docks, noted, "The main building, and the temporary buildings, together constitute a fire-risk that has caused the Hospital Officials and the Bureau [of Medicine and Surgery] much anxiety.... New wards of a permanent character are therefore a necessity, and it is requested that two such wards of fireproof construction be erected."[12] In a letter to the Secretary of the Navy regarding hospital construction on the Pacific Coast, Stitt wrote, "In view of the repeated reports coming from the Naval Hospital Mare Island, as to the great fire risk to patients, ... provisional plans have been prepared that provide a fire-proof hospital to take the place of the present three-story wooden building." Observing the value of the three-story structure as an administrative and therapeutic space, Stitt went on to "recommend carrying out fire-proofing procedures, and in addition,

Part II—The 20th Century

to construct alongside the present hospital, a strictly fire-proof reinforced concrete three-story ward building which could provide accommodations for approximately 200 bed patients.... The wards of the present hospital could then be used solely for ambulatory patients."[13] A few days later, the chief of the Bureau of Yards and Docks authorized preparation of plans to provide fireproof construction not only for bed patients but also for a "psychopathic ward" and a powerhouse. Acting Secretary of the Navy Theodore Roosevelt approved this plan.[14]

In the early 20th century, psychiatrists were called "alienists," a term that comes from the French *aliéniste*, for a physician who treats the mentally ill. In the early days of the naval hospital, mentally ill patients were sent to one of the California "lunatic asylums," either in Mendocino or Napa if their condition suggested possible cure. "Incurables" were transported by train back to St. Mary's Hospital in Washington, D.C., the federal facility operated specifically for their care. As the general patient volume in the Pacific increased and perhaps as a result of lessons learned from World War I (about which more later), the need for a dedicated alienist hospital became clear. Surgeon General Braisted may have been ahead of his local commander in recognizing the need for a psychiatric facility at Mare Island. In a January 1919 endorsement to the Bureau of Yards and Docks (he referred to the bureau as "BuDocks"), he wrote, "The fitting up of a psychopathic ward at this large hospital is considered very necessary," but he added (perhaps in response to a request from Farenholt), "The Bureau does not approve of the installation of the 'padded cell'; this is considered unnecessary and undesirable; the use of padded cells is obsolete."[15] The wheels of naval and congressional bureaucracy moved slowly: it wasn't until 1922 that Surgeon General Stitt wrote to the commandant of Mare Island Navy Yard, "Arrangements have been completed with BuDocks for the construction of a fire-proof building for the care of neuro-psychiatric cases...; this building, however, will not be completed for some time." In October 1923, the chief of the Bureau of Yards and Docks, in an endorsement to the Secretary of the Navy, recommended, "Mare Island— ... At the

Eight. Interbellum

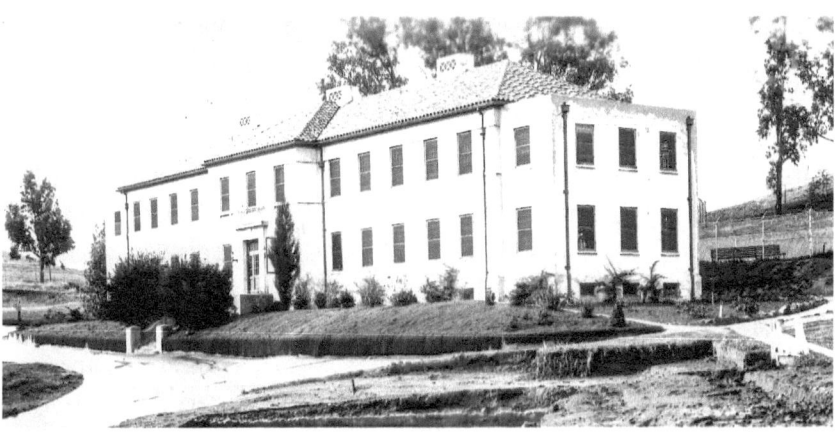

Alienist (psychiatry) building. Official Navy photo, 1928. National Archives, Washington, D.C.

present time, provide ward building facilities of fire proof construction for 200 bed patients; psychopathic ward [underlining mine], power house ... and construction of fire escapes for the present main building, which will be retained for ambulant patients and administrative and commissary purposes."[16]

The care of veterans on behalf of the Veterans' Bureau[17] continued to be a priority of Navy medicine, as reflected in the bureau's report included in the Navy Secretary's annual report for the fiscal year 1922–1923 in which it was noted that the bureau had reserved 160 beds for veteran care and that, beginning in July 1924, 35 of these beds would be at the Mare Island Naval Hospital.

Surgeon General Stitt had one of his assistants, A.W. Dunbar, write a "heads-up" letter to the new hospital commander, C.P. Kindleberger, in May 1925 to prepare him for a visit from Senator Frederick Hale, then a member of the Senate Naval Affairs Committee and therefore influential in affecting Navy-related legislation. Dunbar wrote, "You will find him very much interested in the Naval Hospital and I trust that you will show him that the appropriations for which he has worked so faithfully have been wisely spent." So that you may know the contents of a memorandum given to him, I will quote the paragraph referring to Mare Island:

Part II—The 20th Century

> Under authorization of Congress, the Bureau is proceeding with the erection of a reinforced concrete structure of two wings containing seven wards to replace accommodations in part.... Detached contagious ward and psychopathic ward are also provided for.[18]

Later in the same letter, he wrote, "I understand the psychopathic ward is nearing completion." On June 21, 1926, Kindleberger indeed wrote to the Surgeon General, "The new Psychopathic ward was placed in commission on 17 June 1926."[19] This ward has the distinction of being the first fireproof building completed on the hospital reservation. Built to the latest standards for psychiatric care, the structure provided ample sunrooms for rest and recreation as well as heavy screening over second-story windows to prevent suicides by defenestration.

As noted previously, the bureau planned for and Congress appropriated funds for construction of fireproof structures to accommodate 200 "bed patients." Once again, the wheels turned slowly, but the contract called for the construction of a "double ward building," a sick officers' quarters, a contagious disease ward (another example of science-in-medicine structural symbolism) and a central heating plant, at a cost of $705,000. The *San Pedro [California] News Pilot* reported this on March 24, 1926.[20]

An indication of an emerging element of the "California culture" came in a brief flurry of correspondence in April 1927 in which Kindleberger requested approval to construct additional auto garage and parking facilities. As he put it, "In view of the present custom of two or more cars to a family, it is believed that this improvement is quite necessary." A little later, he wrote to request approval to construct a four-car garage in an unused portion of the nurses' quarters "in view of the increasing number of Nurses quartered in this building who own cars." Remember, this was 1927! Already, the Californians' love of the automobile was manifesting itself. The bureau, ensconced in the stodgy east, was not impressed: "The construction ... is not approved. The Bureau ... considers this project unnecessary."[21]

As if to close out the decade on a high note for the hospital and its patients, Kindleberger announced at the beginning of 1928 that

Eight. Interbellum

as of March 1, patients—except those in the lock ward—would be moved out of the old wood-frame main hospital building to the new ward structure. No more would the staff have to worry about the fire hazard under which they previously labored. Navy medicine on the West Coast had literally moved into the 20th century.[22]

NINE

Into the Great Depression and Then Ramping Up

Researching the hospital history becomes a challenge at this point because, starting around 1930, the once-copious correspondence between the hospital commanders and the Bureau of Medicine and Surgery seems to dry up. I attribute this to the telephone because now, instead of writing to higher headquarters for guidance—this was still the major direction of communication flow; I saw very little "top-down" communication up to this point—it now became an easy matter to simply pick up the phone and call. But this results in a much diminished documentary record. And so, the historian becomes more dependent on newspaper reports. Personal "letters home" would be a wonderful supplement to the historical record, but unfortunately, Americans don't have much propensity to save such materials. One of my recurrent nightmares features the mourning family going through the crate of grandpa's wartime letters and groaning, "Whatever shall we do with these?" then taking the quick and easy solution—the recycle bin!

Now reduced to leafing through the local press,[1] I learned on an almost day-to-day basis how the medical staff integrated itself into the local medical community by hosting specialty meetings. The people of Vallejo and surrounding communities played their part, too, by sponsoring events to provide support and entertainment for hospitalized sailors. The *Vallejo Times-Herald*, the city's morning newspaper, often offers us a more personal look at people and events than we are accustomed to today. For instance, on March 27, 1930, a mid-page headline reports "Farenholt Is New Admiral." The article

Nine. Into the Great Depression and Then Ramping Up

goes on to say that for the first time ever, now there are two officers of this rank on Mare Island—the Navy Yard commandant and the good doctor himself. Farenholt's father, who also had been a Mare Island physician, was the first admiral in that illustrious family; Farenholt Senior died at Mare Island Naval Hospital in 1920.

On July 1, 1930, the paper briefly observed that two doctors, Lieutenants Twitchell and Raines, had reported to the hospital for service as "internes." News of a second elevator for hospital building 71 at a cost of $17,000 was reported in the September 4 number of the press. (A one-sentence paragraph in the October 24, 1931, paper announced that the elevator was now in operation.) On Thursday, October 6, below headlines that a "Converted Mystery Ship Will Sail from Mare Island Today to Appear in a New Fox Picture" was a paragraph describing the monthly hospital fire drill. Reported the *Times-Herald*, "Captain Joseph A Murphy (M[edical]C[orps]) U.S.N. in charge of the hospital, has taken a very active interest in the fire protection of his reservation and has organized the forces at his command so well that it is doubtful if it would ever be necessary for the regular yard department to answer a first alarm there." You must remember that the main administration building and several yard structures were then of wood construction, and so it was altogether appropriate that the hospital commander should be exceptionally fire conscious.

Early in February 1931, there was a brief flurry of correspondence concerning display of the American flag on hospital grounds. You will recall that the earliest images of the new naval hospital featured a flagpole positioned squarely in front of the main entrance. Whereas recollections in the correspondence are vague regarding the history of flag-flying at the hospital, photographic history would suggest that Old Glory (or at least flagpoles), featured prominently from the very beginning. However, in January 1931, Hospital Commander Captain J.A. Murphy wrote to the bureau that the Navy Yard commandant "brought up ... our authority for flying the national colors. He directed [me] to make report and called our attention to Article 323 (3) N[aval] R[egulations]." He went on, "This Article together

Part II—The 20th Century

with Article 1482 (c) N.R. would seem, together with Departmental Letter NH/A3–1 ... to imply that the national ensign should not be flown at the hospital." Looking for a little support in maintaining national pride at the hospital, Murphy closed, "I am writing so that if the Bureau is adverse to removing the colors from this hospital for any reason, you might be able to take action forestalling the Commandant's action." Surgeon General C.E. Riggs's prompt personal reply was brief: "If the Commandant, therefore, objects to the hospital flag and is willing to break down a long standing practice, I do not see how we can very well object."[2] Of the many images of the hospital flagpole I've viewed, none shows the colors flying from it. However, a flag continues to fly from a recently renovated[3] flagpole in front of the main hospital building (H-1).

"Hospital Patients Entertained at Two Recent Events" was the headline of an April 9, 1931, article that described a program sponsored by the Berkeley, California, Red Cross and featuring local dance school and University of California student performances, each of which was "enthusiastically applauded." On Easter Sunday, the Petaluma Red Cross brought "two small girls in cleverly decorated costumes" to distribute Easter eggs and other gifts to the hospitalized men.

Demonstrating that the spiritual needs of hospital patients received attention, the press announced, on December 18, 1931, that by special request, a Christmas cantata would be performed by the First Methodist Church choir at the hospital theater-chapel the following Sunday. The performance was to be followed by a sermon, "The Wise, Wise Men," given by the Rev. Forrest H. Petersime. And on Christmas Eve, Father Muller would celebrate Catholic Mass. This was not solely a spiritual event, as "at the close of the service, coffee and doughnuts will be served in the recreation room."

Entertainment for hospital patients clearly carried high priority. In February 1931 alone, performances by radio stars from Oakland radio station KTAB,[4] an Ancient Order of Foresters ensemble of "16 young ladies," and two famous comedians performing a minstrel show helped relieve hospital tedium.

Nine. Into the Great Depression and Then Ramping Up

A February 26, 1932, *Times-Herald* headline declared, "Hogan Praises M.I. Hospital." The article that followed told about a two-day visit by Van Hogan "[California] department commander of the American Legion." It went on, "Hogan spent considerable time interviewing veterans at the hospital, and found them all pleased with the surroundings and the treatment accorded them."

The hospital also served an educational role for the San Francisco Bay area. In December 1932, the senior dentist, Commander J.W. Crandall, hosted a daylong conference for local dentists. Among the sessions offered were one on modern methods of oral surgery in preparing the mouth for immediate insertion of dentures by Lieutenant (Junior Grade) P.M. Carbiener and one on construction of dentures and new methods for taking impressions. After luncheon, the attendees (including dentists from San Francisco, Palo Alto, St. Helena, Napa, and Vallejo) were given tours of the hospital and of the medical facilities aboard the hospital ship USS *Relief*, then in port.

The December 20 *Times-Herald* noted that holiday entertainment came to hospitalized sailors in the form of a cantata, "The Word Made Flesh," given by a "large chorus" from the Presbyterian church. "The choir, under the leadership of J. Wesley Gebhardt, rendered the numbers in a way which showed the results of masterful training," reported the paper of a performance given at the church a few days earlier.

In a gesture of reciprocity for good deeds by members of the community, the patients of hospital ward 16 each chipped in a "small sum to purchase toys for children of a needy family in Vallejo," reported the *Times-Herald* in its Christmas 1932 edition. The report went on, "An adequate supply of Christmas toys and presents has been purchased and is being used to make the family happy today."

The year-end holidays must have passed quietly at the hospital because the next newspaper coverage didn't appear until February with the headline, "Navy Officer Is Successful in Third Try to Take Life." The young man, a recent Naval Academy graduate, tried to shoot himself while aboard the USS *West Virginia*. His second attempt, according to the newspaper article, occurred in the

Part II—The 20th Century

Mare Island hospital's psychopathic ward, where he stabbed himself 11 times with a pocketknife. Success came when he bolted from a wheelchair while being transported to surgery for repairs of his knife wounds; he threw himself over a third-floor balustrade, landing headfirst on the concrete pavement below.

The Great Depression was said to have had minimal impact on the people of Vallejo because of Mare Island salaries (headline "Navy Payday Puts Coin in Circulation"). "If Vallejo had any worries about its 'cash position' yesterday, they should have been dispelled by the more than $150,000 in cold cash which was paid to officers and enlisted men attached to shore establishments and the 26 ships tied up at Mare Island."[5] Nevertheless, the Navy faced substantial budget cuts of "56 million" according to the April 9, 1933, *Times-Herald*. The potential impact on hospital operations was not detailed in the article.

There was a time when American newspapers wrote the first draft of social history in the form of such pieces as this in the September 30, 1933, *Times-Herald* headline, "Captain Neilson, Family, on Trip":

> A motor tour to the Atlantic seaboard with a stop to visit the Century of Progress fair at Chicago will be started today by Captain and Mrs. John L. Neilson, and their two daughters. Captain Neilson is in command of the naval hospital at the Mare Island navy yard. While in the east they will visit Captain Neilson's mother at Hartford, Conn., and will see relatives of Mrs. Neilson in Washington, D.C. The entire tour will require a month, and they will return by the southern route.

A Thursday, April 12, 1934, entry declared, "Hospital to Open Season April 22: The Mare Island Naval Hospital baseball team will open its 1934 season Sunday, April 22, on the northend diamond at the navy yard against Magistrinis Sporting Good Company. The Hospital expects to have a strong team this season as several star players have been transferred to the island hospital." (I did not follow the team's season in the press.) And on Friday, April 13, "Navy Doctors Play at Local Course: Four Mare Island navy doctors were guests yesterday of the Vallejo Golf Club at the local links. They are

Nine. Into the Great Depression and Then Ramping Up

Dr. Bryan, Dr. Noreen, Dr. F.W. Ryan, and Dr. R.H. Laning." Commander Laning was the hospital chief surgeon.[6]

In Washington, D.C., 1933 saw the inauguration of Franklin Delano Roosevelt and, with that, the arrival of Roosevelt's personal Navy physician, Lieutenant Commander Ross T. McIntire, as White House physician. Roosevelt met McIntire when he was Assistant Secretary of the Navy; he suffered frequent attacks of sinusitis, and his good Navy friend Admiral Cary T. Grayson[7] recommended McIntire as the "best ear, nose and throat man in the Navy." A deep friendship developed, so it was natural that Roosevelt would bring the good doctor with him to the White House. War broke out in Europe when Germany invaded Poland in 1938. From the beginning, Roosevelt understood that despite our nation's neutrality and a strong isolationist sentiment among the citizens, the United States sooner or later would be drawn into the war. Accordingly, he put in place preparations for this inevitability. This included appointing McIntire as Surgeon General of the Navy. "Deep selected" (by the commander in chief), McIntire went from Navy Commander to Rear Admiral in one fell swoop. As we will see, McIntire was an administrative genius.

Hard upon the German invasion of Poland:

> The Surgeon General called a full-dress planning conference immediately, which dealt with necessary expansion in the fields of personnel, logistics, and facilities. An increase in appropriations was an immediate need. The appropriation for BuMed had for some years averaged about $13,000,000 annually, but was about double that amount for fiscal 1939. It was increased to $50,000,000 for fiscal 1940, and rose to about $500,000,000 annually for the later years of the war.[8]

McIntire himself wrote,

> In the first week of September, 1939, I called together the Heads of Departments ... to discuss the events that had taken place in Europe, following the invasion of Poland by Germany. Events that had occurred during the past weeks had convinced me that war was inevitable with Germany and possibly Japan, in the not too distant future. A directive was given at this meeting to all Heads of Departments to prepare an estimate of the situation as far as their Departments were concerned and to present in six weeks, time plans that would be integrated into one overall plan for Medical Department Activities in time of emergency. This was done.[9]

Part II—The 20th Century

Almost simultaneously, on September 8, 1939, President Roosevelt proclaimed a "National Emergency in Connection with the Observance, Safeguarding, and Enforcement of Neutrality and the Strengthening of the National Defense within the Limits of Peace-Time Authorizations." Reserve medical personnel were therefore ordered to active duty. This permitted the "staffing up" of Navy hospitals, carefully planned to meet the estimated need should America go to war.

As war approached, Navy medical planners became well aware of the Mare Island hospital's limitations: its buildings were old, and there was little room for expansion because the hospital reservation was hemmed in to the east by the large and growing industrial portion of the Navy Yard and to the west by hills that rose sharply toward the golf course. Additionally, hospital commanders worried that should an enemy attack the shipyard, the hospital, in such close proximity, might suffer what we today call "collateral damage."

Ten

World War II— Their Finest Hour

On December 7, 1941, the Navy had 19 hospitals in its inventory. Navy personnel abandoned one of these—in Cañacao, Philippines—later that month due to damage caused by Japanese bombing. By the end of the war, the Navy was operating 99 hospitals in the United States and overseas. Patients under the care of Navy medical personnel averaged 7,723 in June 1941, before the war started. In the last year of World War II, that number averaged 90,635.[1]

While naval hospitals had been established in Bremerton, Washington, in 1912, and in San Diego in 1919, at the time of the Pearl Harbor attack, Mare Island was still the most well-developed naval hospital on the West Coast. Even though the hospital commanding officer had recommended ultimate decommissioning of the Mare Island Naval Hospital due to its age, constrained physical space, being hemmed in by the Navy Yard industrial plant, and the risk of inadvertent bombing should an enemy undertake attacks on the shipyard and its ammunition facility, the 12th Naval District Medical Officer, Captain Edward U. Reed, in an October 6 letter to the Surgeon General expressed the opinion that despite these and other concerns, "the four million dollar hospital at Mare Island will be needed for many years, but without further permanent expansion." Reed further indicated that he had already embarked on a search of the San Francisco Bay for a suitable location for a new permanent naval hospital. The Surgeon General concurred with this assessment: "My feeling about the hospital at Mare Island would be that we leave there only facilities sufficient to care for the local personnel."

Part II—The 20th Century

He requested that Reed send him a map with suggested possible hospital locations. This Reed did on November 6, noting, "The best location of [the proposed new] hospital will depend largely on whether the Naval Hospital, Mare Island, California, is to be eventually discontinued as a hospital." McIntire was decisive: on December 12, this telegram appeared:

> DEPT PROPOSES TO CONSTRUCT TEMPORARY HOSPITAL WITH ULTIMATE CAPACITY TO THOUSAND BEDS AND DESIRES DISTRICT TO SELECT SITE PREFERABLY ON HIGHLAND VICINITY OF OAKLAND X SITE SHOULD BE SUITABLE FOR ULTIMATE DEVELOPMENT OF PERMANENT HOSPITAL WHICH WILL LARGELY REPLACE MARE ISLAND HOSPITAL.[2]

Concurrent with this activity, however, Navy authorities had staffed the Mare Island hospital up in anticipation of an influx of casualties, with the call-up of Reserve doctors and nurses. On November 25, 1941, Captain Reed reported, "The Medical Department personnel consists of 56 officers, 50 Nurses and 283 Corpsmen. The staff of medical officers is now adequate in numbers for present needs. The majority of them are Naval Reserve Officers, who are rapidly becoming familiar with Naval procedures."

Inasmuch as the planned naval hospital at Aiwa in Hawaii wasn't yet completed, naval casualties of the attack on Pearl Harbor received their initial care in ad hoc first aid stations, in local clinics and at Tripler Army Hospital. One hundred seventy-nine of these patched-up patients arrived at Mare Island on Christmas Day, 1941.

I remember from my days in training that we used to resent receiving five admissions in the evening, patients admitted for surgery the next day. But the Mare Island staff of doctors, nurses and corpsmen on Christmas Day received 179 of the sickest of patients, many men with severe burns and several with fractures of various bones. One had died of his injuries on his way back to the States. No Christmas deliverance for him, but what a Christmas gift that must have been for the others—back home in the States and in a well-established naval hospital!

Calling up a cadre of Reservists was something of a gamble,

Ten. World War II—Their Finest Hour

and McIntire demonstrated his concern to Captain Reed a week later:

> I hope you will have an opportunity to go to Mare Island shortly after the arrival of the first load of patients from Hawai'i. I want you to be very frank with me as to your opinion of the members of the staff, especially the Reserve officers. We must have no slips in the handling of these cases. Clifton and Dearing [the hospital commanding officer and executive officer, respectively] are excellent men, but I am not so sure of some of the Reserves we are bringing in. They have good reputations but I will feel a lot better about them when I know how they work out.

Ten days after the patients arrived, Reed reported,

> You will be interested to know that 180 patients were recently received from Pearl Harbor and were sent to the Naval Hospital, Mare Island.... The only critical case died on the ship before they reached port. Many of them had extensive burns and there were a number of fracture cases and a few mental cases.... They were handled very well by a detachment of men from the Naval Hospital, directed by Captain Marquette.

Two days later, Captain Clifton, the hospital commander, wrote,

> Captain Reed stated to us that you were somewhat concerned as to whether the reserve officers here could carry on work properly in this hospital during the present emergency.... I have had a chance to observe them under very trying conditions in this short time I have been here, and I feel sure they will bring great credit on the hospital. Dr Dearing is of the opinion they are exceedingly well equipped professionally. As you know on the 25th we had 179 admissions in one day. Many of these cases were badly burned. It was necessary in the wards having burned cases to have as many as seven nurses on duty in each ward. All the medical officers turned to and worked on Christmas day and far into the night and certainly did most excellent work. The spirit shown by them is certainly much to their credit.

He went on,

> This morning [December 29] we have 771 patients of which 735 are sleeping in the hospital and the rest are subsisting at home. We have in the hospital 318 vacant beds that can be used immediately. We have made arrangements with the Yard to take over a barracks which will hold approximately 250 patients.... So unless there is some grave emergency, we are well equipped to take any number of patients from the Pacific area.[3]

Those burn patients received a characteristically innovative Mare Island treatment. The staff dermatologist, Dr. Ralph Pendleton,

Part II—The 20th Century

a Reservist called up from his practice in Salt Lake City, eschewed the standard burn treatment of the day, which called for painting or spraying the burns with a solution of tannic acid. This produced an artificial scab over the burns, protective to be sure but terribly painful when dressings were peeled off to examine the wound underneath. Instead, Mare Island sailors and Marines had their burns sprayed, using a Flit® gun, with a mixture of petroleum jelly (Vaseline®), cod liver oil, and a sulfa antibiotic. This treatment had at least two advantages: it provided instant pain relief, and it left the burns unobscured so that healing could be easily monitored. Moreover, because it did not call for covering the burns with dressings, patients could start full range of motion exercises of burned limbs, important for maintaining their strength and full use.

In October 1942, Hospital Commander A.L. Clifton wrote to Assistant Surgeon General Luther Sheldon, "The representatives of 'Time' and 'Life' Magazines are here ... taking pictures of burns treated by the wax method which we have developed here.... Altogether I think the thing will be a good advertisement for the Medical Department of the Navy." Sheldon replied, "Like you, I think these things when properly done, give the Medical Department desirable publicity." The *Time* article did indeed appear on November 16. It quoted one sailor who had received the treatment, "'We're all taking flit guns of that stuff back to duty,' said a discharged sailor as he packed his bag last week."[4]

Like dermatologist Pendleton, many other Naval Reserve doctors, nurses and corpsmen provided an early and lasting source of staffing as Surgeon General McIntire expanded the Navy's medical forces to meet the demands of the war.[5] One Reservist of particular local interest is Lieutenant Commander Emile F. Holman, MC-V(S), USNR (Medical Corps-Volunteer [Specialist], U.S. Navy Reserve).[6] Holman was the head of the Stanford Medical School Department of Surgery and, at age 51, just two weeks after the attack on Pearl Harbor, volunteered for service despite a long history of opposition to war. Hospital Commander Clifton petitioned the Surgeon General to permit Holman's appointment as chief of surgery at the rank of commander.

Ten. World War II—Their Finest Hour

Holman did indeed serve at Mare Island (I don't know if he was surgery chief, though) but only for 13 months. He added to the Mare Island tradition of innovation by successfully removing a bullet and a piece of shrapnel from the heart muscle of two sailors who'd been wounded during the Pearl Harbor attack—likely the first such surgery ever performed.[7] After that, he served in a succession of base and fleet hospitals and Marine Corps medical battalions as near to the combat as possible, there to apply his particular skills to the benefit of wounded Marines and sailors.[8] After the war, he returned to Stanford, where he continued to write about his wartime experiences for many years.

As we've seen, even before war broke out, the doctors at all levels of leadership were concerned that they have enough facilities and staff for the care of expected casualties. And from the beginning, the wards were crowded. For instance, as early as February 7, 1942, just three months into the conflict, a 12th Naval District inspection reported that the new Contagious Building, with a design capacity of 120, was accommodating 180, made "possible only by putting beds closer together and in solaria, and double deck bunks in the mumps and measles ward, and by quartering patients in basement rooms not intended for that purpose." The inspector noted that the hospital staff consisted of 63 doctors, 169 nurses and 649 corpsmen.[9,10] The May inspection saw that the new four-story ward building (H-81) was finally completed and in use. The sick officers' quarters, "very much overcrowded" with 83 patients—some of whom were living at home—included 16 dependents, though these were soon to be moved to renovated accommodation on the third floor of the original wood-frame hospital building (H-1). He also noted that of the patient census of 1,350, "some 224" were domiciled in non-hospital barracks. This May dispatch also noted for the first time that of the 88 Medical Officers then assigned, 16 were "internes"—that is, trainees. In August, the patient load was now 1,548. Of particular interest was that a blood bank had been established in the new ward building and that while it had just 125 units (pints) of blood, it would be built up to 2,500 units.[11] For the first time, women (Waves) were expected to replace some male hospital corpsmen in the hospital.[12]

Part II—The 20th Century

By February 1943, dependents had been moved to renovated wards on the upper floor of the old H-1. All hospital buildings were now overcrowded, "especially those used for mental cases requiring restraint." Of the hospital's census of 1,858 patients, 540 slept in barracks off the hospital reservation. Staff now included 400 hospital corpsmen of whom 33 were Waves. Quarters for 248 Waves and 54 Waves officers were expected to be completed by the beginning of December.

On November 25, 1942, the new hospital commander, Captain J.P. Owen wrote a "Dear Ross" letter to the Surgeon General to report that he had relieved Captain Clifton.[13] With his staffing and bed capacity situation fairly well under control, Owen seems to have occupied much of his energy to expanding laundry and galley facilities to service the hugely expanded number of patients and staff and to the "Artificial Limb Shop" (informally referred to as the "brace shop") to accommodate the specialists and technicians who were to produce the most advanced prosthetics of the time—this, despite the Surgeon General's declared policy of "no expansion of Naval Hospital Mare Island." A September 1943 inspection report captures the laundry situation pretty clearly:

> Pieces of soiled linen, etc., for the hospital, Yard Dispensary and Yard Dental Clinic averages 163,029 pieces per month or a daily output of 6270 pieces. The hospital average is based on the present patient load. This will increase when the [psychiatric] Unit at Napa is placed in full commission and the WAVE quarters are occupied. It is estimated that this will raise the monthly average by 46,000 pieces.[14]

Commenting on the laundry situation, in another "Dear Ross" letter, Owen noted, "It now takes 3 or 4 weeks to get a shirt or collar from the laundry in this area." Regarding the mess hall situation, the same report noted that staff and patients had to use separate spaces for eating and that patients and junior enlisted corps personnel had to stand in line outside the mess hall, "which is very unsatisfactory in inclement weather." Similarly, the Artificial Limb Shop had sprung up, unanticipated, but needed to be funded and accommodated.[15]

Ten. World War II—Their Finest Hour

Psychiatry at Mare Island

War is the most horrible of human experiences, and descriptions of what we today call PTSD appear as early as the fifth century BCE. Ajax, the protagonist in Sophocles's play of the same name, a Greek hero in the war against Troy, manifests symptoms and behaviors we recognize as those of PTSD. In our Civil War, the symptoms came under the rubric of "soldier's heart"; in World War I, "shell shock" (thought to be a result of the repeated concussions of artillery shells); and in World War II, "combat neurosis" or "combat fatigue."

The American psychiatric community, stung by World War I General John J. Pershing's criticism that not enough was done to screen out soldiers at risk for becoming psychiatric casualties, undertook to avoid the same "error" when the draft was instituted in the late 1930s. Although there was by no means a consensus on this in the psychiatric community, the Selective Service, under the influence especially of Henry Stack Sullivan (director of the William Alanson White Psychiatric Foundation in New York) and Winifred Overholser (superintendent of St. Elizabeth's Hospital in Washington, D.C.), undertook to require screening for the "predisposition" to combat stress reactions. Those deemed vulnerable—about 10 percent of all draftees—were weeded out.[16] But the test of combat quickly demonstrated that in reality no man is "immune" to psychological trauma. Sir Max Hastings, in his excellent one-volume history of World War II (*Inferno: The World at War, 1939–1945* [Vintage Books, 2011]), at one point describes the Australians battling the Japanese in the mountains of New Guinea: it is hot and humid, in an environment crawling with bugs and mosquitoes; clothing literally rots off the soldiers' bodies; food is cold and in short supply. A determined and skilled enemy fights with especial cunning at night. The Aussies battle their way up a mountainside only to be driven back down by determined counterattacks. Under these wretched conditions, Hastings points out, no man is invulnerable to combat stress.

Even in the months before the outbreak of war, both Hospital Commander C.J. Holman and 12th Naval District Medical Officer

Part II—The 20th Century

Reed repeatedly mentioned overcrowding of the Neuropsychiatry Building.[17] Six weeks after the attack on Pearl Harbor, on February 7, 1942, Reed's Mare Island inspection report still noted

> the Neuropsychiatry Building (H-70) is seriously overcrowded, with beds too close together and in the ward solaria and basement. This building has normal accommodation for forty (40) patients and now contains ninety-one (91). This has been especially objectionable during the recent rainy months when outdoor exercise has seldom been possible for these patients.
> Fifty-eight (58) other mental patients are now quartered in a two-story temporary barracks building with double bunks outside the hospital reservation. The transfer of psychotic patients as rapidly as possible to the Veteran's Bureau [sic] or to Washington, D.C. is urgently needed.
> Mental cases should be removed to other hospitals as rapidly as possible.... The Navy Yard is not a suitable place for the handling of mental cases. The noise and frequent alerts and alarms are most disturbing for this type of patient, and accommodations for them should be provided outside the Navy Yard as rapidly as possible.[18]

By the end of May 1942, hospital staff were caring for 237 neuropsychiatry cases, many of whom were quartered in barracks buildings outside the hospital reservation. The most seriously mentally ill—those with psychoses—were being sent to Fort Worth, Texas, in batches of 50, while arrangements had been made to transfer 100 patients to nearby Napa State Hospital.[19] Despite regular transfer of the sickest of patients, neuropsychiatric casualties kept on coming—"We received 16 mental cases from San Diego, and we are getting some from Bremerton..., so they continue to pile up. We are sending a trainload to St Elizabeths[20] on May 14, and we have an additional 50 that we can send to Fort Worth[21] at any time."[22] In November 1942, the Navy approved a supplement to the workforce constructing a new 250-bed facility at Napa State Hospital to speed its completion for use by Navy psychotic patients. Even so, it wasn't until September a year later that the facility opened. The Navy detailed 100 corpsmen to assist in their care at the so-called Imola Annex.

In the meanwhile, Surgeon General McIntire kept looking for places to care for men suffering combat fatigue/neurosis. In March 1943, he asked Owen what he thought about "taking over Sonoma

Ten. World War II—Their Finest Hour

Inn as an adjunct to your hospital." It's not certain how this particular facility, identified as "U.S. Naval Rest Center, Sonoma Mission Inn, Boyes Springs, California," fit into the program. The initiative to establish the rest center came not from the Bureau of Medicine and Surgery but from the vice chief of Naval Operations via the Navy chain of command. In January 1943 correspondence, the chief of Naval Personnel, Admiral Randall Perkins, in establishing this "new station," requested that the Surgeon General allot $225 to it, with an annual allotment of $150.[23] This certainly seems to represent a rather modest gesture of support. Intended for short ("average of 10 days") recuperative stays, the lovely inn, with 200 rooms, appears to have served until war's end but apparently wasn't affiliated with the Mare Island facility.[24]

By 1943, the flow and care of neuropsychiatric patients had settled into a routine: acute cases received a period of treatment and observation wherever they were. Mare Island (on the West Coast) became the center for the care of those deemed to require more extended treatment. Patients could receive care on Mare Island or, for the more severely mentally ill, at the Imola Annex in Napa. Psychotics, the most seriously mentally ill, ultimately would be sent by train or by air to St. Elizabeth's Hospital in Washington, D.C. (officers) or to the Public Health Service Hospital in Fort Worth, Texas. By the summer of 1944, patients deemed to have chronic mental illness could, upon request, be sent to Veterans Administration hospitals near their homes or near relatives.[25]

The diagnosis of PTSD came into official medical use in the late 1970s as psychiatry workers struggled to get an intellectual handle on the phenomenon and then to work out ways to help returning soldiers, Marines and sailors[26] who suffer from it. Once you have a name for something, it's easier to grapple with the issue. When I was in medical school, we cared for a good many World War II and Korea veterans at the nearby Samuel S. Stratton VA Hospital. Many of these men were desperately ill from the effects of chronic alcoholism. They had returned from war and were expected to simply pick up in family, work and social responsibilities right where they left off when they went to war. They didn't receive much medical help or understanding. So, understandably, they reached out to alcohol to numb their psychic pain. We didn't understand much then, and they suffered and died because of it. We understand better now, but people suffering from PTSD still turn to alcohol—and drugs—and they commit suicide. We have a long way to go.

Amputees and the Brace Shop

As Navy combat casualty care became more sophisticated, patients often arrived stateside for definitive care of problems already managed well or for convalescence before being discharged from service or returned to their active units. In the case of amputee care, a Mare Island orthopedist, Lieutenant Commander Douglas D. Toffelmier,[27] took the lead. The story, as related by the official Navy Yard newspaper *Grapevine*,[28] began on Friday, February 19, 1943, with the headline, "'Brace Shop' for M.I. Hospital." As the number of orthopedic casualties increased, Toffelmier became increasingly frustrated by the time it took to obtain properly fitted artificial limbs—then done on contract, a process that could take months from the time bids were opened, contracts awarded, measurements taken and the limbs delivered. So Toffelmier hatched a scheme to open a manufacturing facility at the hospital. The project started small, with materials and manufacturing equipment scrounged from various shops and departments on the Navy Yard. Since the Navy had not anticipated such an activity, there were no funds available to purchase necessary lathes and other equipment. So the doctors went for donations. The first $1,000 came from the workers in Shop 31—the Machine Shop—a Christmas gift to the hospital. Soon thereafter, Delta Theta Tau, a national sorority, pledged $2,000. The same *Grapevine* article told of Toffelmier's intent to train recovering patients in the craft of making artificial limbs, thereby teaching them a craft they could take into civilian life after their discharge from service. "A well known Oakland brace maker (revealed to be Matt Lawrence—'crippled, himself'—in a later article) who has donated his time two or three days

Ten. World War II—Their Finest Hour

each week" would be offered a small salary later on to come to the shop on certain days and teach his trade to men at the hospital. The orthopedist also told the *Grapevine* that he was working on plans to develop a plastic leg that would be lighter than the then-current wooden devices and cheaper—$50 a copy, he estimated, compared with the $250 cost of standard wooden devices. An August 20, 1943, *Grapevine* headline trumpeted, "BRACE SHOP BRINGS M.I. NEW WAR JOB." It went on, "The Naval Hospital Brace Shop, brought into being less than eight months ago with the aid of generous contributions by thousands of Mare Island men and women workers, today won official recognition by the Navy Department." It reported that the Navy Surgeon General had designated the hospital as the official amputation center for the entire Pacific area. By February 1944, Hospital Commander Owen reported, "The artificial Limb Department is improving every week. All the new assistants which the Bureau ordered here to work in the Prosthetic Department are expert mechanics.... We received 7 new amputation cases from the South Pacific today, making a total of 99." That same month, BuMed, in a Navy-wide message, encouraged all Navy medical facilities in the Pacific area to send their amputees, as soon after operation as possible, to the Mare Island hospital to ensure their proper care and training in the use of their artificial limbs.[29]

Local support for the Brace Shop and the hospital was generous. An October 1943 article noted that the Bay Meadows horse racing track, still operating about 20 miles from Vallejo in the East Bay, donated $10,000 in the spring season and had set aside Armistice Day, November 11, as Naval Hospital Day, with proceeds to be divided between the Mare Island and Oakland naval hospitals. Henry Howard Kessler, MD, a specialist in rehabilitation work who volunteered for service in the Navy with the rank of captain, was assigned its director. So famous became the "Brace Shop" that local rumor had it that even royalty were treated here. (I never found documentation of this, however.[30]) One source has the Brace Shop caring for more than 800 amputees at one point during the war. The Amputee Center evolved into the Navy Prosthetics Research Center after the war. The research center worked closely with the Biomechanics Laboratory of the University of California, San Francisco and the University of California (Berkeley) Engineering Materials Laboratory in pioneering work in modern prosthetics. But it all started with "the best prosthetic then known" at the Naval Hospital, Mare Island.[31] The prosthetic work pioneered at Mare Island contributed to the development of modern rehabilitation medicine.

Family Care at Mare Island

The naval hospital was also responsible for the care of Navy wives and children. Navy doctors provided obstetrical care, and there were beds for pediatric cases and adults. Of course, the war expanded the numbers of these patients, too. Captain Reed, the 12th Naval District Medical Officer, wrote to McIntire in March 1943 that since Pearl Harbor, more than 9,000 Navy women and children had been received by the hospitals in the district. This included Mare Island, where much correspondence about upgrades to H-1, the wood-frame structure built in 1900, can be observed. Just before Pearl Harbor, Hospital Commander C.J. Holman received an allotment of $55,000 to open ward space on the third floor of the old hospital.[32] After only a couple of months, the unit was open. Demand was immediate and high. The hospital commander wrote in September 1943 that the new unit had been expanded from 28 to 38 beds and that the hospital stay for maternity cases had been reduced from two weeks to ten days[33] because of the demand for beds.[34] The December 17 *Grapevine* now featured a new separate "Naval Hospital M.I." section, and on this date, the headline was "With Emphasis on Babies." It told of "a nursery large enough to care for over 20 babies" and "a comparatively new incubator, used to care for weak or prematurely born babies." There, the situation apparently stood until the end of the war.[35]

Earlier, I mentioned the generous financial support the hospital received from the community and from the workers of the shipyard.

Ten. World War II—Their Finest Hour

The *Grapevine* regularly reported on more personal support of hospital patients. The Christmas Eve paper reported, under the headline "WARDS FIGHT FOR CHRISTMAS TREE HONORS" (a competition among wards for the best holiday decorations), that "hospitable families of the community" had proffered 260 invitations to patients for Christmas Eve or Christmas Day dinners and parties. In fact, invitations outnumbered available patients—many of whom would be spending the holidays with their own families—by about 2:1. Support came from farther afield, too. A June 1944 "Hospital Scuttlebutt" feature told of three patients being guests of various families in Walnut Creek, 25 miles distant. "They reported a grand weekend." The October 20, 1944, number listed no fewer than three events for several patients in private homes in San Francisco, Lake County and Walnut Creek. Also reported was the appearance of the famous Kay Kyser and his orchestra at the hospital. Several other famous entertainers, including Bob Hope, made appearances, too.

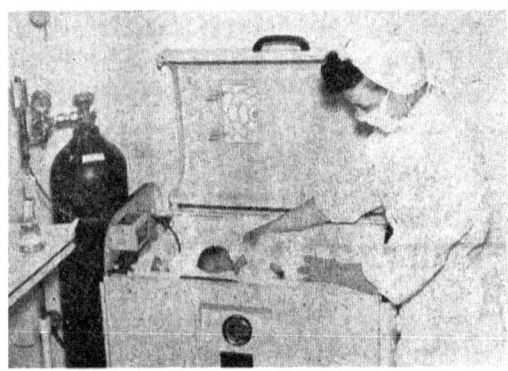

"Shown as she attends a tiny baby in the Castle incubator in the Family Section at the Naval Hospital is Navy Nurse Margaret Phelps, one of the nurses assigned to obstetrical cases." Mare Island *Grapevine*, 17 December 1943. Courtesy the Vallejo Naval and Historical Museum.

Originally designed with a bed capacity for around 600, the hospital at Mare Island grew to a capacity of around 2,300 patients. In today's terms, we would say that the "acuity"—the level of illness—of the vast majority of these men was low: the hospital mainly provided a roof, a bed and three squares a day while they convalesced from illness or injury on their way to discharge or return to duty. Even the amputees were not particularly ill, but they needed expertise in

Part II—The 20th Century

training and a place to stay as they learned how to take care of and use their artificial limbs.

Nevertheless, in their "finest hour," the doctors, nurses and hospital corps personnel dedicated their time and talent to the "repair and rebuilding" of their patients, just as the workers on the shipyard provided invaluable work in building and repairing ships of the Pacific fleet.

ELEVEN

War's End, Immobilization, Korean War, Closure

The end of war resulted in rapid demobilization: patients wanted to go home or to be moved to a hospital nearer to home. Doctors and staff, too, wanted to move back to their prior civilian endeavors. Moreover, from the Mare Island perspective, Navy officials had made it clear they wanted to build another, more modern, permanent hospital "somewhere in the San Francisco Bay area." Accordingly, by August 1946, a year after the war's end, bed capacity was down to 1,000. Consistent with postwar austerity prescribed throughout the services, a series of letters from the bureau directed further reductions in the authorized bed capacity to 750 for 1947, then 700 for 1947 and 1948, and the Surgeon General put a hold on proposed modernization of the operating room suite. The dismal litany of bed capacity reduction continued, to 650 for 1949. In October 1948, Hospital Commander W.H. Perry reported the conversion of prior ward spaces to an upholstery shop, medical library, classrooms and a conference room. He considered these changes "permanent," thereby taking the spaces away from bed capacity.[1]

In August 1949, Perry received notice, via BuMed, from the Veterans Administration Procurement Office that concerning "orthopedic and prosthetic appliances, now being furnished to beneficiaries of the Veterans Administration by the U.S. Naval hospitals at Mare Island, California, and Philadelphia, Pennsylvania. Adequate commercial facilities are now available in both areas, and it is not considered necessary to continue to utilize the services of the Naval Hospitals. Accordingly, notification is given to the effect that Contract VAm-2283 will be terminated, effective September 23, 1949."[2]

In a report to the Secretary of the Navy in February 1950, Surgeon General Swanson noted that Mare Island was "the designated hospital for reception and treatment of neuropsychiatric patients of the Navy from the naval activities and Operating Forces of the Pacific Ocean area and the ELEVENTH, TWELFTH and THIRTEENTH Naval Districts." But this was not to be for long, only "until conversion of suitable security spaces in the U.S. Naval Hospital, Oakland, California, have [sic] been accomplished."[3]

A month later, orders came from the bureau that 174 patients and 8 physicians, 13 nurses and 41 hospital corpsmen were to be moved to Oakland Naval Hospital. The report closed, "Transfer accomplished without incident."[4]

Early 1950 saw the secretary of defense ordering major reductions of domestic military hospital facilities. As a result, the chief of BuMed directed the commanders of naval hospitals at Mare Island and Long Beach to discontinue admitting patients as of February 15. The bed capacity for the Mare Island hospital was set at 50. Nearby naval hospitals (Oakland in the case of the Mare Island facility) were directed to take the patients instead. Patients already in hospital were to be discharged as routine called for. For the moment, military and civilian staffing would be maintained, even as the patient census dropped. Hospital Commander B.W. Hogan replied, in part,

> I certainly deeply appreciate your call and assurance given to me, as the news of the closing of this hospital came as a great disappointment. I had concentrated a year's work in the last three months in the reorganization and improvement of the physical, material, and professional tone of the place and we had just completed plans for submission to the Bureau for renovating the neuropsychiatric buildings; however, I realize the problem is greater than just the local point of view and I am sure that Oak Knoll [Oakland] will be adequately able to take over with little difficulty the neuropsychiatric load as they have locked ward facilities there and should be able to take over the amputee program and shop with no difficulty except the movement of equipment.
>
> The news of the impending hospital closure hit the local community like an atomic bomb explosion, and you may expect to be in for some rough

Eleven. War's End, Immobilization, Korean War, Closure

weather for awhile as the community will fight as a mother tiger defending its young to retain the activity here. They are well organized, have money, and leadership, and there will be protests from various Veterans groups, civic organizations, and from the community as a whole. There is a loss of approximately over $700,000 in civilian pay and over $1,030,000 in military pay for the community. They also feel that it's a bad omen in relation to the activity of the Navy Yard.[5]

And fight it did. Letters from veterans' groups and private citizens flowed in to the Surgeon General's office, sometimes directly, sometimes referred from the offices of Senator Knowland of California and even from the president. In March, Vice Admiral Mahlon Tisdale, probably the most senior retired Navy officer in the area, and once commandant of the Navy Yard, wrote to express his concern about medical support for the community going away. He expressed particular concern about the Brace Shop:

> My main worry now is over the virtual closing of the Mare Island Hospital with the consequent loss of the best amputee center in the country. I am the foster father of the Brace Shop. To me its loss will be a personal tragedy— and a tragedy to the thousands of amputees in and out of the service who benefit by the research being done there.

A reply prepared for Surgeon General Swanson's signature reassured Tisdale that although continued operation of the Brace Shop at Mare Island was not feasible, the full enterprise, including "the experimental work on cineplastics," would be supported at the Oak Knoll facility. In point of fact, an April air mail letter to the hospital commander indicated that the Surgeon General had been given permission by the Under Secretary of the Navy to move the amputation service to Oak Knoll.[6] The record does not indicate the precise date of the move, but subsequent reports of space utilization in the Mare Island complex never again mention the Brace Shop. Thus ends a local story of heroic inventiveness.

The Vallejo Chamber of Commerce long sponsored an "Armed Forces Committee," in reality a very effective lobbying operation. The chief lobbyist was Dr. James Hogan (not related to the hospital commander), whom you will remember from his involvement, as a Navy

Part II—The 20th Century

Reservist, in caring for influenza patients on Mare Island and owner of "Vallejo Central Hospital" in 1918.[7] Hogan's efforts to keep the hospital open were aided by the Korean conflict. Correspondence from the Surgeon General (as chief of the Bureau of Medicine and Surgery) to the chief of Naval Operations at the beginning of June set the active bed count at 100, adding that "complete inactivation of that part of the facility in excess of the authorized bed capacity will be accomplished by 1 July 1950." By the end of July, though, casualties from the United Nations police action were beginning to flow in, resulting in a revised operating bed capacity of 550 to be declared for September. Of these, 500 were allocated to the Army: 200 general medical beds, 200 surgical beds and 100 for neuropsychiatric patients. Shortly thereafter, on the 27th, Camp Stoneman,[8] California, received designation as the Army activity responsible for administrative procedures, with the expectation that "in the near future an Army Administrative Unit will be established at the Naval Hospital to replace the preceding temporary measure." Things moved quickly then, for on September 22, the hospital commanding officer received a phone call from the bureau directing the addition of 300 more beds to be activated, yielding a total of 871. The wartime butcher's bill grew, requiring a total "mobilization capacity" of 972 in November 1950. Thereafter, the need for beds gradually declined again. There things stood until November 1951, when the bed count was revised to 650.[9]

In July 1952, the Surgeon General excerpted a Medical Inspector General's report to the hospital commanding officer:

> The patient load has shown a steady decline over the past several weeks due principally to a decreased number being received from the combat theatre. This is a source of concern to the command because the cost per patient day rises as the census declines and it is feared that should the cost per patient day continue to rise beyond its persent [sic] level of $13.50 orders may be received to again reduce the hospital to an infirmary status. Such an occurrence would be likely to lose permanently the hard core of civilian employees who have once before experienced a loss of their billets due to the five month closure in 1950–51.[10]

The litany continued in a November 1953 Report of Military Inspection forwarded by the Navy Yard commandant (now

Eleven. War's End, Immobilization, Korean War, Closure

designated as "Commander, Mare Island-Vallejo Area, U.S. Naval Base San Francisco") up the chain of command:

> As of the inspection date the patient-count at Naval Hospital, Mare Island was 301 as compared with an average daily census of 425 for the current calendar year. The low figure as of the inspection date represents a steady trend since the cessation of Korean hostilities. This low patient count results in a relatively high per-patient cost of operation.

His report also laid out another problem being faced by all military services—the flight of doctors:

> The medical officer situation of the Armed Forces is reflected in the staff changes at the Naval Hospital, Mare Island. On 1 October 1952 there were 47 medical officers on board and during the past 12 months 34 medical officers were received, 27 medical officers transferred, *23 medical officers separated from the service* and 24 medical officers remaining [emphases mine]. There are only 4 medical officers aboard who were present one year ago. It is obvious that the most effective use cannot be made of a staff of medical officers with the excessive turnover.[11]

The next correspondence about bed capacity came in this letter from Vice Admiral Tisdale to Captain Clarence Brown, the Deputy Surgeon General, in August 1953. It's revealing in many regards, as is the cryptic reply from Brown:

> I had had no inkling that the census of patients had dropped so low. I guess the Chamber of Commerce had been lulled into lethargy by the continued existence of the Police Action in Korea. Someone on the street stopped me to say the census is down to barely over 200; and that there are no Army or Air Force patients. The latter surprised me, as I had heard so much Washington talk about unification of the Medical services[12] that I had supposed it had been started in a modest yet practical way. However, all of that is just surmise, and is down stream. My interest now is to find out as much as I can properly repeat about the prognosis for continuation of a hospital here. I start my "chataqua circuit" of reports about the county on the 14th. I know I will have the question thrown at me; and I would like to appear as wise as is practicable. It may miss me till Sunday the 15th, when I address the Masonic breakfast club at Mare Island. I feel sure it will be tossed in my lap then. Please let me know whatever you properly can. If your reply may not reach me by the 15th please wire me collect.
>
> I have noted that the House reversed itself in appropriating for out-patient (so to speak) Veteran beds. According to my information this means that there will be money for 5,086 more veteran beds—both in and

Part II—The 20th Century

out patient—than there was last year. Do you have any idea of reestablishing a modest veterans section at Mare Islands [sic]. As you know, this is a Critical Defense Area with many veterans living in it. I am told the ambulance trip to Oak Knoll is $35.[13]

Brown was less wordy in his wired reply of August 15:

> YOUR 9 AUGUST, OUR CURRENT PLANS RETAIN HOSPITAL IN STATUS QUO. FURTHER REDUCTION OF CENSUS MAY GENERATE ATTEMPTS TO FORCE CLOSURE. NAVY AUTHORIZED HOSPITALIZE VETERANS ONLY ON REQUEST OF VA. NONE REQUESTED FY 54.

Note the "none requested FY 1954."[14] The VA wasn't asking for beds; there was no operational reason to keep the hospital open.

A memorandum from the assistant secretary of the Navy for Air to the assistant secretary of Defense for Health and Medical Affairs in August 1954 pretty well captures thinking regarding the Mare Island hospital:

> Relative to our discussion of the merits of improving the Mare Island Hospital rather than the Oak Knoll Hospital, I have looked into the subject, and the following are the facts:
>
> The U.S. Naval Hospital at Mare Island is a 772-bed hospital of which the average patient census is 350. The building is 30 to 35 years old [sic], is in the center of the industrial area of the shipyard, and there is no room for expansion. In addition, it is in an undesirable location.
>
> On the other hand, the Naval Hospital at Oak Knoll contains 3,247 beds with an average census of 1,300 to 1,500 patients. It is approximately 10 years old, of WW II construction, located in the hills overlooking Oakland, and has plenty of room for expansion. It is more centrally located with respect to all the Naval activities of the Bay area and has better accessibility than the Mare Island Hospital.
>
> Therefore, our decision, with which I must concur, was to concentrate on improving the Oak Knoll Hospital rather than the smaller, older one in the shipyard at Mare Island.[15]

Post–World War II–authorized bed count peaked at 959 in October 1955. The 12th Naval District Medical Officer noted that the hospital was servicing military personnel from the Navy base and nearby Travis Air Force Base, as well as a large retired and dependent population living in Vallejo and the Napa Valley. He also pointed out that an average of 52 babies were born per month.

Eleven. War's End, Immobilization, Korean War, Closure

Secretary of the Navy Notice 5450 of February 17, 1956, titled, "U.S. Naval Hospital, Mare Island, Vallejo, California; established status and change of mission of" declared, under "Mission," that henceforth, the naval hospital would "provide limited general clinical and hospitalization service for the shore activities and fleet units present in the Mare Island Shipyard. General clinical and hospitalization services in a limited degree will also be provided for dependents of the Armed Services and other authorized supernumeraries in the vicinity of the Naval Shipyard. The operating capacity will be 50 beds."[16]

The commanding officer wrote to the Surgeon General on October 11, 1956,

> It is expected that additional funds will be required in the amount of approximately $2,500,000 per quarter ... in order that civilian specialists, including pathologist, radiologist and ophthalmologist may be employed on a part time basis. Since the transfer of Medical Officers with these specialties, it is believed that adequate patient care can not be given without the services of such specialists.

This indicates one of the complications of running a hospital on a "skeleton" staff: you have to "hire in" specialist care.[17]

In reply to an April Fools' Day 1957 letter from California congressman John F. Baldwin (Sixth Congressional District California, including Vallejo) to the chair of the House Appropriations Committee advocating for retention of the Mare Island facility based on the economy of retaining it versus building a new hospital at Oak Knoll, Deputy BuMed Chief Rear Admiral Bruce E. Bradley, citing the bureau's March 28, 1957, letter to the Secretary of the Navy, replied,

> The Navy has been vitally concerned for a number of years with the proper siting of a modern hospital in the San Francisco Bay Area. The Dallerup Committee recommended to the Secretary that a complete and impartial study for future naval hospital requirements in the San Francisco Bay Area be carried out. As a result of this committee's recommendation, a study taking into consideration all factors was accomplished by the architectural firm of Skidmore, Owings and Merrill in September 1955 at a cost of $90,000. This study recommended that a single facility be constructed on the present site of the Oakland Hospital.
> The present facilities at Mare Island are now approximately 35 years old

Part II—The 20th Century

[sic] and would require extensive repairs, alterations and modernization to meet the partial future bed requirements in the San Francisco Bay area. This hospital is hemmed in by industrial facilities. Adequate space does not exist to provide for the construction required to meet the total 1500-bed requirement of the San Francisco Bay Area. Consequently, construction of a second naval hospital equally as large would be required to meet the total patient load in the area.

It has been previously determined that it is uneconomical to operate two large naval hospitals in this area. The mission of the U.S. Naval Hospital, Mare Island, was reduced approximately one year ago in accordance with this concept.

The surgical suite and other ancillary facilities at Mare Island would require extensive, major, costly repairs to meet present and future standards for the best medical care. Provisions for newer methods of treatment, such as radioisotopes, cannot be economically incorporated in the Mare Island hospital plan.

The Department of Defense is in agreement with Navy plans for construction of a new hospital on the Oakland site. These plans have been co-ordinated with hospital construction of the other two military services.

The location of Mare Island is not as convenient to the majority of patients. It is not well situated for railroad and commercial air evacuation; and in case of war or catastrophe, the hospital is more easily isolated. In addition, the Mare Island hospital is in a relatively inaccessible location to the medical consultants whose services are an essential requirement for the successful operation of a large naval teaching hospital.

There are no plans at present to reactivate the U.S. Naval Hospital, Mare Island, over the 50 bed capacity now authorized.[18]

Never daunted, the congressman wrote to the Honorable Secretary of the Navy Thomas S. Gates on May 20, 1957, suggesting that the Neuropsychiatry Service and/or the Amputee Center be returned to its "home" at Mare Island. He argued that its proximity to Napa State Hospital was a benefit. Rear Admiral B.E. Bradley, Acting Surgeon General of the Navy, replied on the Secretary of the Navy's behalf, in a detailed and compelling rebuttal,

> First, it must be pointed out that no one service in a naval hospital is a separate unit unto itself. All services complement or are dependent upon other services and all are part of the whole. To separate one from the other causes inefficiency, increases the cost, and multiplies the administrative procedures.
>
> Both the neuropsychiatric service and the orthopedic service, of which the amputee center is a part, are approved by the Council on Medical

Eleven. War's End, Immobilization, Korean War, Closure

Education and Hospitals of the American Medical Association and the individual Specialty Boards for residency training in these specialties. One reason for this approval is that the services are part of a large general hospital and there is close liaison with civilian medical consultants at nearby hospitals and with the facilities of the University of California. It is considered highly unlikely that this approval would be granted if the two services were transferred to the Mare Island hospital. The residency training program is one of the most important factors in building and maintaining the high standards of Navy medicine as it is today.

The amputee center with its brace and limb shop has achieved world acclaim. It is part of the orthopedic service and could not be separated from it without causing serious deterioration of the orthopedic training program. The majority of skilled workers in the brace and limb shop live in the general vicinity of the Oakland hospital and work closely with the University of California on various projects. The patients treated in the amputee center are long-term patients and, in many cases, require the use of other services in the hospital.

Therefore, due to the serious impairment of the residency training program, the costs involved in moving the two services and in the repair and modernization necessary, the Bureau of Medicine and Surgery does not consider it feasible to transfer the neuropsychiatric service or the amputee center from the U.S. Naval Hospital, Oakland, to the U.S. Naval Hospital, Mare Island.[19]

Frank B. Berry, MD, Assistant Secretary of Defense for Health and Medical Affairs, further replied to Congressman Baldwin on July 9, 1957,

> I promised you I would make further inquiries as to the hospital at Mare Island. Admiral [Bartholomew W.] Hogan [the Surgeon General] informs me that Mare Island has become a high cost operation and that the Bureau of Medicine and Surgery recommended its inactivation....
>
> I asked him to consider particularly the hospitals in the immediate vicinity of Vallejo. He has submitted the following list: The Kaiser Foundation Hospital of 334 beds in Vallejo. The Vallejo [General] Hospital of 654 beds is also there. Nearby at Napa there is the Parks Victory Memorial Hospital and in Berkeley, only 10 miles away, there are three hospitals of about 475 beds capacity total. From the military standpoint there is the Travis Air Force Base Hospital on one side, Hamilton Air Force Base Hospital on the other side and the large Oakland Naval Hospital. As you are aware, this is a part of the Naval program of general retrenchment and from a letter I have from Admiral Hogan and from a personal interview with him, it seems to me this will have very little impact on the hospital situation in Vallejo.[20]

Part II—The 20th Century

On the very same day, Captain Evan C. Stone, Jr., MC, USN, director of Planning Division BuMed, wrote to Senator William F. Knowland on July 9, 1957,

> Inadequate funding during 1957 had to be compensated for by drastically reducing the program for equipment replacement for repairs to the physical plant of naval hospitals....
>
> In addition to the foregoing requirements, this Bureau is faced with the unbudgeted requirement of $775,500 for a new influenza vaccine to combat the threat of the spreading influenza epidemic from the Far East.... It was determined that none of the Bureau of Medicine and Surgery programs or functions could be feasibly eliminated in order to satisfy the budgetary cut.
>
> The compound effect of the present reductions together with the fundamental stringency of the 1958 budget and the impact of heavy unbudgeted requirements necessitated serious action. Accordingly, the Department of the Navy proposed closure of the naval hospitals at Corona, California, and Mare Island, California, as the only feasible method by which the accumulative financial problem facing the Bureau of Medicine and Surgery can be alleviated and an effective, efficient medical care program be conducted throughout the rest of the Navy.[21]

On July 17, in a sad last-minute effort, newspaper owner and powerful local figure Luther Gibson telegraphed Surgeon General Bartholomew W. Hogan, only recently the Mare Island Naval Hospital commander, "VERY MUCH CONCERNED WITH ANNOUNCEMENT THAT MARE ISLAND HOSPITAL WILL BE CLOSED.... I WILL APPRECIATE TALKING WITH YOU BY PHONE ABOUT THE HOSPITAL IF YOU WILL CALL ME COLLECT AT TIMES-HERALD, VALLEJO."[22] A headline in the *Vallejo News-Chronicle* agreed, the next day declaring, "Closing of M.I. Hospital Called 'Decided Mistake.'"

Chief of Naval Operations Arleigh Burke even weighed in on the matter, perhaps indicating just how much gravitas this Navy town carried then. After citing facts and arguments already discussed, he closed, "You may be assured, Senator [Kuchel of California], that the decision to close the Naval Hospital at Mare Island has not been an easy one to make."[23]

The headline struck in the October 15 *Vallejo Times-Herald*: "Corona, M.I. Hospitals Told to Stop Accepting Patients":

Eleven. *War's End, Immobilization, Korean War, Closure*

The Navy is sending out directions to the Mare Island ... hospital not to accept patients after Aug. 15 except on an emergency basis. On Sept. 15 after the patient load has contracted, they will start moving the patients and expect to have all the patients moved by Oct. 15. A few people will stay about two weeks at the hospitals in order to properly secure the place.

Thus, with the strokes of many bureaucratic pens did the Navy's first West Coast hospital meet its end after an illustrious career marked by intrepidity and innovation.

Epilogue

But Navy medicine did not leave Mare Island. Concurrent with hospital closure, a clinic was opened on the first floor of the sick officers' building, and the hospital commanding officer's home was razed to create space for a clinic parking lot. In about 1989, the Navy opened a futuristic new clinical structure in the light industrial portion of the Navy Yard, away from the hospital compound. With the closure of the Navy Yard in 1996, control of the clinic fell to the Department of Veterans Affairs.

About five years after the hospital closed, the buildings were taken over by the U.S. Navy Schools Command, the Navy's main educational establishment. The Schools Command expanded from H-1 to 32 structures over 48 acres on the yard. It was succeeded by the U.S. Navy Combat Systems Technical Schools Command (CSTSC).

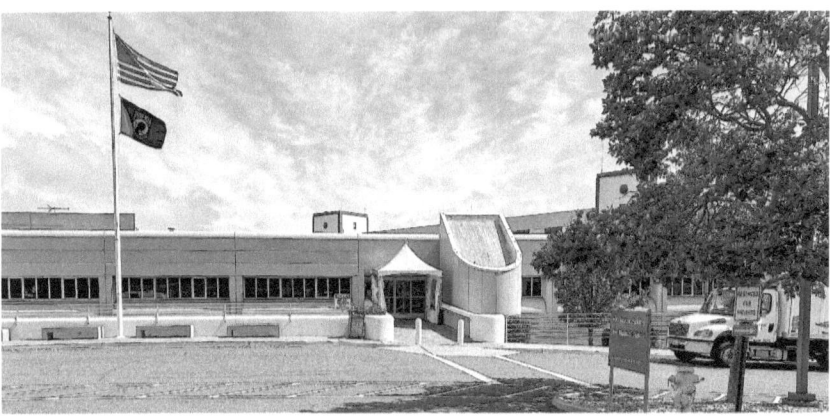

The last Navy medical facility on Mare Island, now a Department of Veterans Affairs outpatient clinic. Photograph by the author.

Epilogue

With the motto "Potestas est scientia" (Knowledge is power), these schools trained a couple of generations of sailors and specialty officers in the operation and maintenance of a huge variety of electronic systems used by the Navy. In the lead-up to the Navy base closure, the CSTSC closed its doors in 2005 and moved its headquarters to San Diego. I have argued, without any clear evidence whatever, that U.S. information/cyber warfare got its start in the hallowed halls of the former naval hospital.

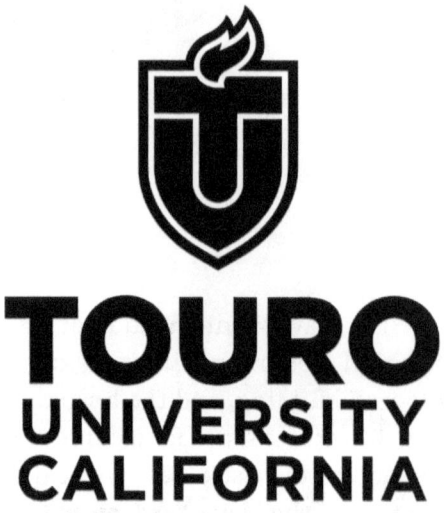

Touro University Logo. Courtesy Touro University California.

In 1999, Touro University California, a division of Touro University of New York City, moved from temporary quarters in San Francisco to Mare Island. The university owns 23 buildings on 44 acres of the former hospital compound. It currently uses three buildings for instructional space and at least two others for administration. The university offers degrees in osteopathy (DO), pharmacy (PharmD), nursing (MS, FNP, Psychiatric Nursing), education (MA, PhD), public health (MPH), and sonography (AA), as well as a dual degree for physician assistants (PA/MPH). The student body stands at about 1,300, with a faculty of around 100.

Thus, future health professionals now tread the hallowed grounds once traversed by our nation's war heroes, informed, one may hope, by the same Mare Island tradition of innovation and intrepidity.

Epilogue

Naval Hospital, Mare Island, Officers in Charge and Commanding Officers

Station Hospitals, 1855–1871

USS WARREN (STATION HOSPITAL), 1855–1857
Officers in Charge:
Asst. Surgeon John Mills Browne, 1855–1857

USS INDEPENDENCE (STATION HOSPITAL), 1857–1861
Officers in Charge:
Surgeon John S. Messersmith, 1857–1859
Surgeon Washington Sherman, 1859–1861

Temporary Hospital, 1861–1871

Officers in Charge:
Surgeon William S. Bishop, 1861–1865
Surgeon John Mills Browne, 1865–1868
Surgeon William E. Taylor, 1868–1871

Naval Hospital, Mare Island, 1871–1904

Officers in Charge:
Surgeon George W. Woods, 1871–1872
Medical Inspector Jacob S. Dungan, 1872–1875
Medical Inspector James Suddards, 1875–1876
Medical Inspector John Mills Browne, 1876–1880
Medical Inspector George Peck, 1880–1883
Medical Inspector Somerset Robinson, 1883–1886
Medical Director Albert L. Gihon, 1886–1888
Medical Director Adrian A. Hudson, 1888–1890
Medical Director Newton L. Bates, 1890–1892
Medical Director George W. Woods, 1892–1897
Medical Director George P. Bradley, 1897–1900
Medical Director James A. Hawke, 1900–1903
Medical Director Manly H. Simons, 1903–1904

Epilogue

Naval Hospital, Mare Island, 1904–1957

Commanding Officers:
Medical Director Manly H. Simons, 1904–1906
Medical Director Remus C. Persons, 1906–1909
Medical Director Manly H. Simons, 1909–1911
Medical Director Phillips A. Lovering, 1911–1913
Medical Director Manley F. Gates, 1913–1916
Medical Director Thomas A. Berryhill, 1916–1917
Medical Director Ammen Farenholt, 1918–1921
CAPT Thomas A. Berryhill, MC, 1921–1924
CAPT Charles P. Kindleberger, MC, 1924–1928
CAPT Ammen Farenholt, MC, 1928–1930
CAPT Joseph A. Murphy, MC, 1930–1931
CAPT John L. Neilson, MC, 1931–1934
CAPT W. Neil McDonnell, MC, 1934–1938
CAPT Edward U. Reed, MC, 1938–1940
CAPT Charles J. Holman, MC, 1940–1941
CAPT Alfred L. Clifton, MC, 1941–1942
CAPT John P. Owen, MC, 1942–1945
CAPT Clarence W. Ross, MC, 1945–1948
CAPT Wendell H. Perry, MC, 1948–1949
CAPT Bartholomew Hogan, MC, 1949–1950
CAPT H.V. Packard, MC, 1950–1953
CAPT Thomas Hays, MC, 1953–1956
CAPT Paul K. Perkins, MC, 1956–1957
CAPT Cecil H. Coggins, MC, 1957

Chapter Notes

Preface

1. "To be a Reservist is to be 'Twice a Citizen'—Churchill" was emblazoned high on the bulkhead of the drill hall in the Navy Reserve Center on Treasure Island in San Francisco Bay, one of the many places I performed weekend drills during my 24-year Navy Reserve career. It's not at all certain Churchill uttered those words, but the attribution has been repeated beyond counting.

2. David Glasgow Farragut is revered in the Navy. The famed naval officer David Porter adopted the young Farragut, who then served under him, at age 11, during the War of 1812. At age 12, he commanded his first ship, the captured Royal Navy HMS *Barlay*. In 1856, you will learn as you read this book, he founded the Navy's first West Coast shipyard at Mare Island. His fame skyrocketed with his naval victory in the Civil War Battle of Mobile Bay, where he is said to have shouted the words, "Damn the torpedoes. Full speed ahead!" to encourage his fleet into battle. As a result of his victory there, Farragut was the first American officer to receive the rank of rear admiral. He continued to serve, rising to the rank of admiral, until he died at age 69.

3. Cutler, D.W., and Cutler, T.J. (eds.), *Dictionary of Naval Abbreviations, Sixth Edition* (Annapolis: Naval Institute Press, 2005).

Introduction

1. By long tradition, naval physicians rate the sobriquet of "surgeon," whether they are in fact surgeons or not. The term "Medical Officer" is a more modern usage. While physicians in the Navy are still referred to generically as "surgeons," the term "doctor" is used in informal conversation—"Good morning, Doctor Jones," except for commanders and above, where the rank is used—"Good morning, Captain Snyder." "Doc" is an honorific applied, with deepest respect, only to enlisted medical personnel, corpsmen. To this day, the British express medical ranks thus—"surgeon commander," etc.; not so in the American navy, where, in formal discourse, only the military "commander," etc., is used.

2. Snyder, T.L., "There's the Medical Corps and the Dental Corps and the ..." (part 3 of a five-part series on the Navy's nine "corps" of which five are medical), *Of Ships and Surgeons* (November 20, 2020 blog post), https://ofshipssurgeons.wordpress.com/2020/11/20/theres-the-medical-corps-and-the-dental-corps-and-the-part-3-of-a-5-part-series-on-the-navys-nine-corps-of-which-five-are-medical/.

3. Retief, F., and Cilliers, L.P., "The Influence of Christianity on Medicine from Graeco-Roman Times up to the Renaissance," *Acta Theologica*, 26(2) (2006): 220, 221, https://www.medievalists.net/2016/01/the-influence-of-christianity-on-medicine-from-graeco-roman-times-up-to-the-renaissance/.

4. Risse, G.B., *Mending Bodies, Saving Souls: A History of Hospitals* (Oxford: Oxford University Press, 1999), 79.

Notes—Chapter One

5. Savage-Smith, Emilie, "Hospitals," in *Islamic Culture and the Medical Arts* (Bethesda: National Library of Medicine, 1994). An online version of a brochure to accompany an exhibition in celebration of the 900th anniversary of the oldest Arabic medical manuscript in the collections of the National Library of Medicine, https://www.nlm.nih.gov/exhibition/islamic_medical/index.html#toc.

6. Smith, T., "The Knights of Saint John and the Hospitals of the Latin West," *Speculum*, 3(4) (1978): 709–733, https://www.journals.uchicago.edu/doi/epdf/10.2307/2849782.

7. Risse, G.B., "Medicalization: Hospitals Become Sites of Medical Care and Learning" (2004) [unpublished manuscript], https://www.academia.edu/10342059/Medicalization_Hospitals_Become_Site_of_Medical_Care_and_Learning. Professor Risse appears to have coined this term.

8. Mann, W.L., "The Origin and Early Development of Naval Medicine," *United States Naval Institute Proceedings*, 55(319) (1929): 772ff, https://www.usni.org/magazines/proceedings/1929/september/origin-arid-early-develop ment-naval-medicine.

9. Langley, H.D., *A History of Medicine in the Early U.S. Navy* (Baltimore: Johns Hopkins University Press, 1995), 8.

10. Langley, 79–102.

11. Langley, 284–289.

12. Lott, A.S., *A Long Line of Ships: Mare Island's Century of Naval Activity in California* (Annapolis: U.S. Naval Institute Press, 1954). I read Lott's research notes in the National Archives. He did not leave a list of his sources.

13. Lott, 235.

14. Lemmon, Sue, *Closure: The Final Twenty Years of Mare Island Naval Shipyard* (Vallejo, CA: Silverback Books, 2001), 377.

Chapter One

1. This wasn't the end of the story. While the "Oregon Treaty" of 1846 settled the border on the mainland, the maritime border between Vancouver Island (British) and "the (U.S.) mainland," an area that contained several navigable waterways, was left vague. A local dispute between British subjects and U.S. citizens on San Juan Island led the United States to send troops to occupy the island while the Brits positioned warships offshore. Although the disagreement never escalated beyond heated feelings, a settlement of the conflict, arbitrated by Germany's Kaiser Wilhelm I in 1872, confirmed the border, with San Juan Island in U.S. territory.

2. Until the first decades of the 20th century, every American navy yard featured a receiving ship. These were obsolete vessels, dismasted and covered over and more or less permanently anchored close to shore. They acted as an administrative center for the yard. Mare Island's receiving ship, USS *Independence*, was the Navy's first major warship, launched in Charlestown (Boston) Navy Yard in 1814. The ship was anchored at Mare Island from 1857 until 1912.

3. Hagan, Kenneth J., *This People's Navy: The Making of American Sea Power* (New York: Free Press, 1991), 118–120.

4. Lott, 7.

5. Farragut had deep maritime roots. His father was a Spanish merchant captain who shipped the lad off to live with Navy Captain David Porter "to learn a trade." He joined the Navy at age 10, and by age 12, he commanded a prize ship captured in the War of 1812. Having proven his abilities repeatedly, Farragut early rose to positions of responsibility, and so it was only natural that he would be sent to the West Coast to establish the new Navy Yard. I gleaned the broad outline of Farragut's career from the American Battlefield Trust. https://www.battlefields.org/learn/biographies/david-g-farragut.

6. Lott, 9–10.

Notes—Chapter Two

Chapter Two

1. The fourth U.S. warship bearing the name USS *Warren*, a second-class sloop-of-war, was built at the Boston Navy Yard and commissioned in 1827. Her initial battles came while protecting merchantman convoys against pirates in the Mediterranean.

2. Hamersly, L.R., *The Records of Living Officers of the U.S. Navy and Marine Corps*, 3d ed. (New York: J.B. Lippincott, 1878), https://babel.hathitrust.org/cgi/pt?id=uc1.%24b41417&seq=205.

3. Commander David Farragut, Commandant, to Secretary of the Navy James C. Dobbin, June 15, 1855. Records of the Bureau of Yards and Docks, RG 71 (Letters Received from Commandants, Mare Island, August 11, 1884–December 28, 1857), Box 50, Entry 5, 8. National Archives Building, Washington, DC [hereafter NAB].

4. A "spirits ration"—half pint of distilled spirits or one quart of beer—was part of Navy fare until the Civil War, when Congress discontinued it in 1862. Private stocks of liquor were permitted on board ship, however, until Secretary of the Navy Josephus Daniels prohibited it by General Order 99, effective July 1, 1914. Alcohol consumption is not allowed aboard U.S. Navy ships (except under special conditions and only then with permission of the Commanding Officer and the Medical Officer or Medical Department representative [usually a senior corpsman]). To this day, a cup of Navy coffee is referred to as a "cup of Joe" in sarcastic honor of Josephus Daniels's General Order 99.

5. Surgeon John S. Messersmith to Chief of the Bureau of Medicine and Surgery William Whelan January 15, 1857, Letters Received (Letters from All Sources), January 1857–February 1886, p. 79. Records of the Bureau of Medicine and Surgery, RG 52, Entry 7, Box No. 1, NAB.

6. Surgeon William S. Biship to Whelan, April 1, 1863, RG 52, Entry 1, Box 80, pp. 1–6, NAB.

7. Water issues were a continuing concern in terms of quantity and quality.

8. A Hospital Fund to provide for the relief of sick and disabled merchant seamen was established by Congress in 1798. It required the deduction of 20 cents a month from their wages for this purpose. Congress extended the fund to Naval officers, seamen and Marines in 1799. The Naval Fund was made separate in 1811.

9. Whelan to Bishop (date not recorded), Records of the Bureau of Medicine and Surgery, RG 52, Entry 1, Correspondence 1842–1941; Letters Sent, September 1842–February 1886, Volume 24, 604–605.

10. A prescient comment: the permanent hospital wouldn't be opened until 1871, eight years on.

11. Navy Yard Commandant Captain T.O. Selfridge to Chief of the Bureau of Yards and Docks Admiral Joseph Smith, June 8, 1863. Records of the Bureau of Yards and Dock, Letters and Telegrams Sent to the Bureau of Yards and Docks, RG 181, Entry 166, Box No. 1, Volume 1, p. 68, National Archives and Records Administration—Pacific Region (San Francisco) [hereafter NARA–Pacific Region (SF)].

12. Bishop to Whelan, July 1, 1863, RG 52, Entry 7, Letters Received (Letters from All Sources), Box 18, July 1863, 3, NAB.

13. Surgeon David Harlan [USS *Saranac*] to Surgeon William Bishop, July 1, 1863, 4, RG 52, Entry 7, Box 18, July 1863, NAB.

14. Admiral Joseph Smith to Selfridge, July 6, 1863. Records of Mare Island Navy Yard 1854–1940. Letters Received from the Bureau of Yards and Docks, November 1855–December 1892; November 1895–July 1965, RG 181, Entry 65, Box 2, Larger of 2 Volumes, July 6th 1863. NARA–Pacific Region (SF).

15. Smith to Selfridge, August 13, 1863.

16. This arrangement satisfied neither the local Navy authorities—who feared that sailors sent to San Francisco would

Notes—Chapter Two

simply disappear—nor the sailors themselves—who didn't cotton to being hospitalized in the company of merchant mariners, whom they saw as an inferior lot.

17. Bishop to Whelan, October 19, 1863, RG 52, Entry 7, Letters Received, Box 21, October 1863, 347, NAB.

18. Cormack, Joseph M., *The Legal Tender Cases—A Drama of American Legal and Financial History* (Williamsburg, VA: William and Mary Faculty Publications, 1929), 1497, https://scholarship.law.wm.edu/facpubs/1497. Prior to 1862, most financial transactions in the United States were paid in "specie"—either silver or gold coin. By 1862, the U.S. government had run out of gold with which to finance the Civil War despite the flow of California gold into the national economy. Desperate to pay soldiers and sailors and pay for supplies, and realizing that to increase taxes or issue bonds would take too much time in a period of immediate need, the government resorted to printing paper money—"legal tender." At the time of issuance, a dollar in gold could buy $1.21 in legal tender. At its worst, in July 1864, a paper dollar was worth about $0.35 in gold. Ellison, Joseph, *California and the Nation 1850–1869* (New York: Da Capo Press, 1969). This is a reprint of the original article which appeared in *Publications in History*, vol. XVI, Berkeley, University of California Press (1927). The California Constitution prohibited the creation and circulation of paper money inside the state, and gold was the "main staple commodity" of the state. Californians were accustomed to the jingle of metallic currency in their pockets. The U.S. Supreme Court, in several decisions after the Civil War, appeared to back Californians' right to their metallic currency for transactions inside the state. Nevertheless, the California treasurer astutely converted gold collected from Californians for payment of federal taxes to legal tender and netted for the state treasury about a 7 percent profit on the arbitrage.

19. Selfridge to Whelan, November 21, 1863, RG 52, Entry 7, Letters Received, Box 22, 287, November 1863, NAB.

20. Bishop to Whelan, January 6, 1864, RG 52, Entry 7, Letters Received, Box 24, January 1864, 139, NAB.

21. A cutting out expedition involves "rescuing" a ship that's under control of, for instance, pirates. These risky actions were undertaken to return stolen ships (and hopefully their cargoes and crews) to their rightful owners.

22. One of the surgeons in attendance was Platon Vallejo, MD, a son of the last Mexican governor of California, Mariano Guadalupe Vallejo. Reputedly the first Californio (Californian of Hispanic lineage) to graduate from a North American medical school—others presumably were educated in Mexico or Spain—Vallejo graduated from Columbia Physicians and Surgeons in New York City. Local tradition holds that Platon graduated second in his Class of 1864, but the medical school alumni office told me in a phone conversation that Columbia had a pass/fail system in those days, with no letter grades. But they said his graduation thesis, on the secretions of the kidneys, won second prize that year. Vallejo served as an Army surgeon during the Civil War. After a short stint as surgeon for the Pacific Steam Packet Company, a shipping firm, he settled into a long and distinguished practice in Vallejo, California, retiring in his 80s.

23. Case Paper and Form X regarding "Charles B. Scott, Seaman received July 12, 1870, from USS *Mohican*. Diagnosis by Hospital Ticket, gunshot wound (left hip). Was wounded during an attack on a piratical vessel." RG 52, Entry 25, Records of the Bureau of Medicine and Surgery, Headquarter Records, Medical Journals and Reports on Patients, Hospital Tickets and Case Papers, 1825–1889, Mare Island 1868–1870 [sic], Box 25, Vol. dated 1871.

24. The Sanger Plan, named for "Civil Engineer of the Navy" William P.S. Sanger, according to the National Park Service, provided for a naval hospital. Historical American Buildings Survey,

Notes—Chapter Three

National Park Service Department of the Interior Washington, D.C. 20240 HABS No. CA-1543 HABS No. CP,-154.3 ADDENDUM TO: Mare Island Naval Shipyard Mare Island Vallejo Solano County California, http://lcweb2.loc.gov/master/pnp/habshaer/ca/ca2500/ca2540/data/ca2540data.pdf.

25. Wylie, W.G., *Hospitals: Their History, Organization and Construction* (Orlando: D. Appleton, 1877), 213. "In 1863, the Boston Free City Hospital was partly built. The original plan consisted of a grand central administrative building, connected with six widely-detached, three-story pavilions by curved, one-story corridors. Only two of the pavilions of the old plan were erected."

26. Whelan to Bishop, September 19, 1863, RG 52, Entry 1, Correspondence 1842–1941; Letters Sent ("Letter Book"), September 1842–February 1886, Vol. 17 (page not recorded), NAB.

Chapter Three

1. Horwitz to McArthur, June 2, 1866, 336.
2. Horwitz to McArthur, June 18, 1866, 379.
3. Horwitz to McArthur, July 11, 1867, vol. 35, 331.
4. Horwitz to McArthur, July 22, 1867, 371.
5. Horwitz to Craven, July 26, 1867, 385.
6. *Message from the President of the United States to the Two Houses of Congress at the Commencement of the Third Session of the Fortieth Congress with the Reports of the Heads of Departments and Selections from Accompanying Documents* (1869) (Washington, D.C.: Government Printing Office, 1869), 737–738, https://books.google.com/books?id=gMxDMQEp8YMC&printsec=frontcover&source=gbs_ge_summary_r&cad=0#v=onepage&q&f=false.
7. Horwitz to McArthur, September 21, 1868, Vol. 37, 311.
8. McArthur to Horwitz, September 29, 1868, RG 52, Records of the Bureau of Medicine and Surgery, Entry 7, Letters Received, Box 68, 1868, Letter Book 9.
9. McArthur to Horwitz, February 9, 1869, RG 52, Entry 7, Box 70, 1869, Letter Book 1, 90.
10. Horwitz to Browne, January 18, 1869, RG52, Entry 1, Letters Sent, Vol. 38, 64.
11. Horwitz to Browne, February 13, 1869, 53–54.
12. Acting Mare Island Commandant Werden to Horwitz, March 19, 1869, RG 181, Letters, Telegrams to the Bureau of Medicine and Surgery 9-[18]63-01-1907, Box 1, Vol. 2, 4.
13. Commandant Craven to Horwitz, June 18, 1869, RG 52, Entry 7, Letters Received, Box 72, 1869 May–June 1869, 99.
14. Craven to Horwitz, June 25, 1869, RG 52, Entry 7, Box 72, May 1869–June 1869, 283.
15. Horwitz to McArthur, June 3, 1869, RG 52, Entry 1, Vol. 38, 277.
16. "Regional Note: Low, swampy land is *tules [too-lees]* or *tule [too-lee]* land in the parlance of northern California. When the Spanish colonized Mexico and Central America, they borrowed from the native inhabitants the Hahuatl word *tollin*, 'bulrush.' The English-speaking settlers of the West in turn borrowed the Spanish word *tule* to refer to certain varieties of bulrushes native to California. Eventually, the meaning of the word was extended to the marshy land where the bulrushes grow." *American Heritage Dictionary of the English Language* (4th ed.) (Boston: Houghton Mifflin, 2000), 1854.
17. Surgeon Browne and Mare Island Civil Engineer Calvin Brown to BuMed, August 2, 1869, RG 52, Entry 7, Box 73, 1869, Letter Book 8, August, 7.
18. Browne to the BuMed, July 21, 1869, RG 52, Entry 7, Letters Received, Box 73, 1869, Letter Book 7, 358.
19. Brown to the BuMed, August 12, 1869, RG 52, Entry 7, 1869, Letter Book 8, 115.
20. 0.07 inches—1.78 mm—thick.
21. Parker, Harry (ed.), *Kidder-Parker*

Notes—Chapter Four

Architects' and Builders' Handbook, Eighteenth Edition (Hoboken: Wiley, 1942), 437. Information faxed to the author compliments of the Linda Hall Library of Science, Engineering and Technology, Kansas City, Missouri.

22. Browne to BuMed, August 2, 1869, RG 52, Entry 7, Box 73, 1869, Letter Book 8, 7.

23. Browne and Brown to BuMed, September 6, 1869, RG 52, Entry 7, Box 74, 1869, Letter Book 9, 52.

24. Browne and Brown to the Bureau of Medicine and Surgery, October 12, 1869, RG 52, Entry 7, Box 74, 1869, Letter Book 10, 224.

25. Browne and Brown to BuMed, November 9, 1869, RG 52, Entry 7, Box 75, 1869, Letter Book 11, 97.

26. Lott, 101.

27. Browne and Brown to BuMed, May 28, 1870, RG 52, Entry 7, Box 78, 1870, Letter Book 5, 218.

28. Browne and Brown to BuMed, December 3, 1869, RG 52, Entry 7, Box 75, 1869, Letter Book 12, 28.

29. Browne to the Bureau of Medicine and Surgery (BuMed), January 29, 1870, RG 52, Entry 7, Box 76, 1870, Letter Book 1, 401.

30. Bureau of Medicine and Surgery (BuMed) to Browne, February 10, 1870, RG 52, Entry 1, Vol. 39, 150, NAB.

31. Browne and Brown to BuMed, February 9, 1870, RG 52, Entry 7, Box 76, 1870, Letter Book 2, 69.

32. Browne to BuMed, May 21, 1870, RG 52, Entry 7, Box 78, 1870, Letter Book 5, 181.

33. Surgeon General Wood to Browne, June 1, 1870, RG 52, Entry 1, Vol. 39, 278. Wood is the first chief of the Bureau of Medicine and Surgery to also carry the title of Surgeon General of the Navy.

34. Browne to BuMed, March 8, 1870, RG 52, Entry 7, Box 77, 1870, Letter Book 3, 88.

35. BuMed to Browne, April 4, 1870, RG 52, Entry 1, Vol. 39, 221.

36. Browne to BuMed, April 7, 1870, RG 52, Entry 7, Box 77, 1870, Letter Book 4, 123.

37. Browne and Brown to BuMed, May 21, 1870, RG 52, Entry 7, Box 78, 1870, Letter Book 5, 181.

38. Browne and Brown to BuMed, May 28, 1870, RG 52, Entry 7, Box 78, 1870, Letter Book 5 (page not recorded).

39. Browne to BuMed, July 7, 1870, RG 52, Letters Received, Box 79, Entry 7, 1870, Letter Book 7, 21.

40. BuMed to Browne, September 21, 1870, RG 52, Entry 1, Vol. 39, 387.

41. BuMed to Browne, November 23, 1870, RG 52, Entry 1, Vol. 39, 445–6.

42. Browne to BuMed, August 8, 1870, RG 52, Entry 7, Box 79, Entry 7, 1870, Letter Book 8, 102.

43. BuMed to Browne, August 18, 1870, RG 52, Entry 1, Vol. 39, 363.

44. Note that nurses are paid less than the chief cook. Nurses then were male—the first female nurse would arrive sometime later.

45. These were "Naval Hygiene, Braithwaite's Retrospect [of Medicine], Physician's Monitor, Medical Record & National Medical Journal."

46. Browne to BuMed, August 19, 1870, RG 52, Entry 7, Box 79, Entry 7, 1870, Letter Book 8, 196.

47. Browne to BuMed, August 29, 1870, RG 52, Entry 7, Box 79, Entry 7, 1870, Letter Book 9, 270.

48. Browne to BuMed, October 1870, RG 52, Entry 7, Box 80, Entry 7, 1870, Letter Book 10, 104.

49. Woods to Goldsborough, November 23, 1870, RG 52, Entry 1, Vol. 39, 445–6.

50. BuMed to Browne, December 22, 1870, RG 52, Entry 1, Vol. 39, 464.

51. My wife Gina, who grew up in Hazleton, the heart of Pennsylvania coal country, assures me that anthracite—hard—coal from the Scranton region is the hottest and cleanest burning of coals.

52. BuMed to Browne, December 24, 1870, RG 52, Entry 1, Vol. 39, 465.

Chapter Four

1. *Evening Chronicle*, Vallejo (California), Wednesday, February 1, 1871, Page

Notes—Chapter Four

1, Column 5. Microfilm, John F. Kennedy Library, Vallejo, California. USS *Saginaw* was the first ship built at Mare Island in 1859. A side-wheeler, the ship plied the far reaches of the western Pacific on several missions. The ship was shipwrecked on Kure Atoll, near Midway, in 1870. The story of the crew's rescue is an epic tale.

2. Mare Island Shipyard Log, February 1, 1871, RG 181, Records of Naval Districts and Shore Establishments, Mare Island Naval Shipyard, Office of the Commandant, Shipyard Logs, 1859–1946, from 12/27/1870-1/17/1872 (NS-S, accession number 181-95-020, Box 9, Vol. "M. I. #00558," 37. NARA–Pacific Region (SF) [San Bruno].

3. Surgeon Browne to BuMed, February 5, 1871, RG 52, Entry 7 ("Letters from All Sources"), January 1857–February 1885, Box 82, 1871, Letter Book 2, 49.

4. Surgeon Browne to BuMed, February 5, 1871, 220.

5. The rainy season in Northern California generally runs from November through April. Typically, no rain whatsoever falls from May through October.

6. Browne to BuMed, 1871, RG 52, Entry 7, Box 52, Letter Book 2, 174.

7. BuMed to Browne, May 17 and July 1, 1871, RG 52, Records of the Bureau of Medicine and Surgery, Headquarters Records, Correspondence 1842–1941, Letters Sent, Entry 1 ("Letter Book") September 1842–February 1886, Vol. 40, "Letter Book 41," May 17, 1871, 9 and July 1, 1871, 53.

8. Surgeon G.W. Woods to BuMed, November 1871, Entry 7, Box 86, 1871, Letter Book 11, 215.

9. Woods to BuMed, December (date not recorded) 1871, RG 52, Letters Received, Entry 7, Box 87, 1871, Letter Book 12, 132.

10. BuMed to Browne, February 2, 1872, RG 52, Entry 1, Vol. 40, Letter Book 41, 236.

11. Browne to BuMed (date not recorded) 1877, RG 52, Letters Received, Entry 7, Box 121, 1877, Letter Book 8, 168.

12. Browne to BuMed, December 7, 1877, RG 52, Letters Received, Entry 7, Box 123, Letter Book 12, 72.

13. BuMed to Brown (date not recorded), RG 52, Letters Sent, Entry 1, Vol. 42, Letter Book 43, 65.

14. Hospital Officer in Charge (OiC) Medical Inspector Somerset Robinson to BuMed, December (date not recorded) 1883, RG 52, Letters Received, Entry 7, Box 174, 1883, Letter Book 12, 84.

15. A flat-bottomed boat used for transport of goods and personnel.

16. Hospital Officer in Charge (OiC) Medical Inspector Somerset Robinson to BuMed, December (date not recorded) 1883, RG 52, Letters Received, Entry 7, Box 174, 1883, Letter Book 12, 116.

17. Navy Yard Commandant J.H. Russell to BuMed, May (date not recorded) 1884, RG 52, Letters Received, Entry 7, Box 178, 1884, Letter Book 5, 103.

18. Robinson to BuMed, September (date not recorded) 1884, RG 52, Letters Received, Entry 7, Box 180, Letter Book 8, 154.

19. Robinson to BuMed, September (date not recorded) 1884, RG 52, Letters Received, Entry 7, Box 180, Letter Book 9, 170.

20. BuMed to Robinson, September 26, 1884, RG 52, Letters Sent, Entry 1, Vol. 45, Letter Book 46, 131.

21. BuMed to Hospital Officer in Charge Albert L. Gihon, May 1888, RG 52, Entry 11, Box 15, File 2885B. This is a large packet of correspondence concerning the hospital water supply that spans the dates June 20, 1887, through May 22, 1888.

22. Gihon to BuMed, August 31, 1888, RG 52, Entry 11, Box 22, file dated August 31, 1888.

23. Medical Director Arian A. Hudson to BuMed, November 6, 1888, RG 52, Entry 11, Box 24, file dated November 6, 1888.

24. Browne to Secretary of the Navy William E. Chandler, August (date not recorded) 1889, RG 52, Entry 11, Box 29, File 2239.

25. Browne to the Secretary of the Navy, October 1889, RG 52, Entry 11, Box

Notes—Chapter Four

30, File 2660, NAB. This is also available on page 8 of a digital copy of the report at https://books.google.com/books?id=i43QotxmIRYC&printsec=frontcover&source=gbs_ge_summary_r&cad=0#v=onepage&q&f=false.

26. Woods to the Bureau, date not recorded, RG 52, Entry 11, Box 55, File 758, NAB.

27. Green Valley Falls is a hilly wooded area about 25 miles north-northeast of the city of Vallejo, California.

28. Woods to BuMed, July 11, 1895, RG 52, Entry 11, Box 72, File 6340, July 11, 1895.

29. Browne to BuMed, date in 1870 not recorded, RG 52, Entry 7, Box 79, 1870, Letter Book 7, 21.

30. Woods to BuMed, date not recorded, RG 52, Entry 7, Box 85, 1871, Letter Book 9, 14.

31. BuMed to Woods, RG 52, Entry 1, "Letters Sent," Vol. 40, Letter Book 41, 105.

32. BuMed to Woods, RG 52, Entry 1, 290.

33. Hospital Officer in Charge Joseph S. Dungan to BuMed, July 5, 1872, RG 52, Entry 7, Box 90, 1872, Letter Book 7, July 5, 97.

34. I commented on the "gold coin" matter in the first chapter. During the Civil War, the Union government took the national currency off the gold standard. California remained a gold standard state, and almost all transactions in California were paid in gold coin or, if in the (devalued) national "legal tender," at a premium of 10–40 percent over the nominal value of the paper money.

35. Dungan to BuMed, July 20, 1872, RG 52, Entry 7, Box 91, Letter Book 8, July 20, 1872, 218.

36. Hospital Officer in Charge George Peck to BuMed, May 12, 1881, RG 52, Entry 7, Box 153, File 178.

37. I searched, unsuccessfully, for the use of "felt" in relation to gas lighting. I suspect the writer here intended the term "mantle," which is a small mineral-mesh bag suspended over the gas outlet. The burning gas heats the mantle which then produces a bright light.

38. Peck to BuMed, May 26, 1881, RG 52, Entry 7, Box 153, File 410.

39. Peck to BuMed, September 9, 1881, RG 52, Entry 7, Box 156, File 97.

40. Peck's Submission for Naval Estimates October 1881, RG 52, Entry 7, Box 157, 1881, Letter Book 10.

41. Peck to BuMed, June 27, 1882, RG 52, Entry 7, Box 162, 1882, Letter Book 6, 266.

42. Peck to BuMed, August 18, 1882, RG 52, Entry 7, Box 164, 1882, Letter Book 8, 182.

43. BuMed to Peck, August 29, 1882, RG 52, Entry 1, Vol. 43, Letter Book 44, 343, 29.

44. Peck to BuMed, September 16, 1882, RG 52, Entry 7, Box 164, 1882, Letter Book 8, 149.

45. Peck to BuMed, date not recorded, RG 52, Entry 7, Box 164, 1882, Letter Book 8, 205. Undated but presumed to be September 21, as the document lies between two others of that date.

46. Surgeon General Phillip S. Wales to Peck, September 23, 1882, RG 52, Entry 1, Vol. 43, Letter Book 44, 353.

47. Wilson is identified as president of the Vallejo Gas Light Company in 1886 correspondence. RG 52, Entry 11, Box 13, File 1428B.

48. E.B. Wilson to Surgeon General Wales, October 19, 1882, Entry 7, Box 165, 1882, Letter Book 10, 274.

49. Peck to BuMed, December 18, 1882, RG 52, Entry 7, Box 166, 1882, Letter Book 12, 198.

50. Peck to BuMed, August 4, 1883, RG 52, Entry 7, Box 172, 1883, Letter Book 8, 56.

51. BuMed to Peck, August 11, 1883, RG 52, Entry 1, Vol. 44, Letter Book 45, 108.

52. Vallejo Gas Light Company to BuMed, September 26, 1883, RG 52, Entry 7, Box 172, 1883, Letter Book 9, 305.

53. Somerset Robinson to BuMed, November 19, 1883, RG 52, Entry 7, Box 172, 1883, Letter Book 11, 185.

54. BuMed to Navy Yard Commandant J.H. Russell, November 27, 1883, RG 52, Entry 1, Vol. 44, Letter Book 45, 187.

Notes—Chapter Four

55. Russell to BuMed, February 5, 1884, RG 52, Entry 7, Box 176, 1884, Letter Book 2, 62.

56. Russell to BuMed, February 14, 1884, RG 52, Entry 7, Box 176, 1884, Letter Book 2, 150.

57. BuMed to Russell, February 21, 1884, RG 52, Entry 1, Vol. 44, Letter Book 45, 269.

58. Hudson to BuMed, Entry 11, Letters to and from the Bureau of Medicine and Surgery, Box 26, March, April 1889.

59. RG 52, Entry 11, Box 43, File 1415 "Received Sep 22, 1891"; this file contains all correspondence related to the construction of the new hospital commander's residence. The report mentioned is dated October 7, 1891; all contents in the file are arranged chronologically.

60. Woods to BuMed, July 18, 1892, RG 52, Entry 7, Box 48, in File 758, Received June 20, 1892, File 941, Received July 25, 1892.

61. A modern 15-watt incandescent light bulb produces roughly 18 candle-power. Extrapolated from the formulation that "a 100 W incandescent light bulb emits about 120 cd" [cd = candela; 1 candela = 1 candle-power], found at http://en.wikipedia.org/wiki/Candela.

62. Woods to BuMed, 28 June, 1892, RG 52, Entry 7, Box 48, File 773, Received July 5, 1892.

63. Woods to BuMed, date not recorded, received October 10, 1892, RG 52, Entry 7, Box 48, included in File 1348.

64. Speaking tubes were installed in naval vessels up through the 1950s. They required no maintenance and, after the development of the telephone, served as a backup system in the event of power failure during combat. In the hospital, one can imagine an attendant on the second floor yelling through the tube to the steam boiler operator in the basement, "We need more heat up here!"

65. Browne to BuMed, February 4, 1879, RG 52, Entry 7, Box 130, February–March 1879, 1879, Letter Book 2, February.

66. Hospital Director Jacob S. Dungan to BuMed, August 29, 1872, RG 52, Entry 7, Box 91, 1872, Letter Book 8, 326.

67. Economic History Association, eh.net, https://eh.net/encyclopedia/history-of-the-u-s-telegraph-industry/.

68. Browne to BuMed, February 4, 1879, RG 52, Entry 7, Box 130, 1879, Letter Book, 2, File 32.

69. Browne to BuMed, June 5, 1879, RG 52, Entry 7, Box 132, May–June 1879, 1879, Letter Book 5, 38.

70. Gihon to BuMed, June 27, 1879, RG 52, Entry 11, Box 15, File 2885B.

71. Woods to Surgeon General James R. Tryon, March 21, 1896, RG 52, Entry 11, Box 74, File 7313, February 18, 1896 (contains File 25466, March 21, 1896, Woods to Bureau).

72. Strictly speaking, the hospital was not "under the command" of the Navy Yard commandant. The hospital as well as the Marine Corps barracks and the Ammunition Depot were "tenant commands" of the Navy Yard; they could almost be looked on as renters of territory there. The relationship of the Navy Yard commandant to the hospital commander would be roughly similar to that of a landlord and tenant and not as a commander—subordinate one.

73. Laryngoscope—a device for looking into the larynx (voice box) by way of the mouth; endoscope—any device for peering into a body cavity, be it an ear canal or a rectum.

74. Woods to Tryon, February 4, 1897, RG 52, Entry 11, Box 84, File 31428, Woods to Surgeon General, via Commandant of the Yard.

75. See Chapter 1.

76. Woods to Surgeon General James C. Palmer, December 11, 1872, RG 52, Entry 7, Box 87, December 1871–January 1872, 132.

77. Dungan to BuMed, July 9, 1872, RG 52, Entry 7, Box 90, June 1872–July 1872, 169.

78. Suddards to Surgeon General Joseph Beale, August 16, 1875, RG 52, Entry 7, Box 109, 1875, Letter Book 8, August, 183ff.

79. Browne to BuMed, May 29, 1879, RG 52, Entry 7, Box 132, 1879, Letter Book 5 May, Entry 31.

Notes—Chapter Four

The hospital must have been most unhealthful, especially on hot summer days. It's surprising that the simple plumbing expediency of "siphon traps," a commonplace today, had not been utilized during hospital construction, especially since such devices have been described as early as a century before. The toilets ("water closets") that were installed originally were of a "pan" design. In essence, the toilet bowl was suspended over a pan-shaped device that, when closed, formed the bottom of the bowl. After using the toilet, the user activated a lever which simply dropped the pan, and the bowl contents dropped into a straight pipe that led to the sewer. Unless the seal between the pan valve and toilet bowl was perfect (apparently a rare occurrence), smells from the sewer passed freely back up the pipes and into the hospital halls and rooms.

80. 226,338, Patented April 6, 1880, http://www.google.com/patents/US226338.

81. Navy Yard Commandant E.R. Colhoun to Civil Engineer C. Brown (with copy to Surgeon General Phillip Wales), October 27, 1880, RG 52, Entry 7, Box 148, 1880, Letter Book 10, October, Entry 512, October 27.

82. Peck to Wales, September 1, 1881, RG52, Entry 7, Box 156, 1881, Letter Book 9, September, Entry 12.

83. Peck to Wales, October 1, 1881, RG 52, Entry 7, Box 157, 1881, Letter Book 10, October, Entry 32.

84. Peck to BuMed (Telegram), October 30, 1881, RG 52, Entry 7, Box 157, 1881, Letter Book 10, October, Entry 3, 419.

85. In the 19th century, asphaltum—we would call it "tar" today—was found in many California locations, not the least of which La Brea Rancho near Los Angeles. The Fourth Annual Report of the (California) State Mineralogist (for the year ending May 15, 1884) describes the manufacture of asphaltum pipes thus: "In 1870–71, asphaltum pipe was manufactured by J.L. Murphy, at his works on King Street, San Francisco, by coiling burlap, after being passed through a trough filled with melted asphaltum, on a wooden mandrel [spindle] covered with paper to facilitate its removal. Any desired thickness and strength could be given to the pipe by regulating the length of the cloth in proportion to the size of the pipe required.... When taken off the mandrel the pipes were glazed inside, by stopping up one end, pouring in some melted asphaltum and then rolling them rapidly on a table, the superfluous material flowing out at the open end. The table was covered with coke dust, a portion of which adhered to the outside of the pipe, forming a smooth, dry, and hard coating. The pipe was light, durable [sic], and cheap." https://books.google.com/books?id=Vs23AAAAIAAJ&pg=PA291&lpg=PA291&dq=asphaltum+pipes&source=bl&ots=B1TXNAqqmV&sig=2ncBeA6GGsC8Y5OYJSOeQIKDla4&hl=en&sa=X&ved=0CCAQ6AEwAWoVChMI87vI9bmiyAIVkpWICh296gp1#v=onepage&q=asphaltum pipes&f=false.

86. Peck to Wales, December 2, 1881, RG 52, Entry 7, Box 158, Letter Book 12, December 1881, Entry 15.

87. Peck to Wales, September 26, 1882, RG 52, Entry 7, Box 164, August–September 1882, 238.

88. Peck to Wales, January 15, 1883, RG 52, Entry 7, Box 167, January 1883, 256, NAB.

89. Navy Yard Commandant, Rear Admiral G.E. Belknap to Surgeon General Gunnell, May 27, 1887, RG 52, Entry 11, Box 15, Entry 2720B, Received June 3, 1887.

90. By way of a "refinement," in November 1886, Surgeon Gihon reported, "I ... inclose [sic] requisition for one case of water closet paper [we call it toilet paper] to prevent choking of valves, and traps, which is now of almost daily occurrence [sic], through the use of stiff paper, pasteboard, rags and other improper materials." In 1889, Surgeon Hudson noted, "Herewith I enclose open purchase requisition for toilet paper for use in this hospital. In explanation of the frequency of requisitions for this article, I desire

Notes—Chapter Four

to state that owing to the obstructions which have occurred in the drains at various times I thought it best to supply the general closets [toilets] of the building with this paper, in place of newspapers which have heretofore been used." Sailors were a tough lot in those days! Gihon to BuMed, November 16, 1886, RG 52, Entry 11, Box 12, Entry 1020B, Received November 16, 1886; Hudson to BuMed, June 11, 1889, RG 52, Entry 11, Box 28, Entry 1851, Received June 18, 1889.

91. Bates to BuMed, February 10, 1892, RG 52, Entry 11, Box 46 [1892], File 207, Received February 17, 1892.

92. Browne to Commandant Rear Admiral J. Irwin, April 4, 1893, RG 52, Entry 11, Box 55, File 884.

93. Woods to Browne, April 29 and May 8, 1893, Box 55, Entry 11, File 1195.

94. Browne to BuMed ("Form W"), February 5, 1871, RG 52, Entry 7, Box 82, 1871, Letter Book 2, 49.

95. Browne to BuMed, February 27, 1871, RG 52, Entry 7, Box 82, 1871, Letter Book 2, 226, NAB.

96. Browne to BuMed, March 8, 1871, RG 52, Entry 7, Box 83, March 1871 and June 1871; April and May 1871 not located, 1871, Letter Book 3, 89.

97. Lott, 102.

98. Mare Island Shipyard *Grapevine*, August 21, 1962.

99. Dungan to BuMed, August 29, 1872, RG 52, Entry 7, Box 91, Letter Book 8, August 1872, 234ff.

100. Dungan to BuMed, August 29, 1872.

101. U.S. Department of Commerce, Bureau of the Census (1949), *Historical Statistics of the United States, 1789–1945* (300), U.S. Government Printing Office, http://www2.census.gov/prod2/statcomp/documents/HistoricalStatisticsoftheUnitedStates1789-1945.pdf.

102. Dungan to Surgeon General Joseph Beale, June 1, 1874, RG 52, Entry 7, Box 102, 1874, Letter Book 6, June, 148.

103. Dungan to Beale, June 18, 1874, RG 52, Records of BuMed, HQ Records, Correspondence, Letters Received ("Letters from All Sources") January 1857–February 1885, Entry 7, Box 102, 1874, Letter Book 6, June, 148.

104. Medical Inspector James Suddards to Beale, August 23, 1875, RG 52, Entry 7, Box 109, 1875, Letter Book 8, August, 246.

105. Alta California, Vol. 29, No. 9802, February 7, 1877, http://cdnc.ucr.edu/cgi-bin/cdnc?a=d&d=DAC18770207.2.44&e=-------en--20--1---txIN--------1.

106. Personal: "The Russian Navy and Mare Island, 1862–2009" (unsigned, not dated) cited in a personal communication by Barbara Davis, librarian at the Mare Island (Vallejo, California) Historic Park Foundation Museum, from its collection, September 16, 2015.

107. Browne to BuMed, January 16, 1877, RG 52, Entry 7, Letters Received, Box 117, 1877, Letter Book 1, January, 206 and 296.

108. Browne to Surgeon General William Grier, February 12, 1877, RG 52, Entry 7, Letters Received, Box 118, 1877, Letter Book 2, February, 92.

109. Browne to Grier, May 21, 1877, RG 52, Entry 7, Box 119, 1877, Letter Book 5, May, 188.

110. "The Russian Ball," headline in *Alta California*, 29(9829) (March 6, 1877), http://cdnc.ucr.edu/cgi-bin/cdnc?a=d&d=DAC18770306.2.34&e=-------en--20--1---txIN--------.

111. Peck to Wales, July 9, 1881, RG 52, Entry 7, Box 155, 1881, Letter Book 7, July, Entry 197.

112. Wales to Peck, August 3, 1881, RG 52, Vol. 43, Letters Sent, September 1842–February 1886, Vol. 43, Letter Book 44, 119.

113. Peck to Wales, September 26, 1882, RG 52, Entry 7, Box 164, August–September 1882, 1882, Letter Book 9, September, 238.

114. Peck to BuMed, August 4, 1883, RG 52, Entry 7, Box 172, August–September 1883, 1883, Letter Book 8, August, 55.

115. Peck to BuMed (Telegram), August 10, 1882, RG 52, Entry 1, Letters Sent, Vol. 40, May 1871–February 1886, Vol. 46.

Notes—Chapter Four

116. Gihon to Gunnell, October 27, 1886, Entry 11, Box 12, Entry 934B, November 4, 1886.

117. Gihon to Gunnell, November 1, 1886, RG 52, Entry 971B, Box 12, November 9, 1886.

118. Woods to Surgeon General James R. Tryon, August 15, 1893, RG 52, Entry 11, Box 58, File 2522, Received August 22, 1893.

119. Suddards to Beale, August 14, 1875, RG 52, Entry 7, Box 109, 1875, Letter Book 8, August, 158.

120. This is notable. Joseph Lister published his first papers demonstrating a marked reduction in infections after surgery by the use of carbolic acid sprays in the operating room in 1867. MacCormac was an early advocate of the Listerian technique, and his textbook on the procedure appeared just 13 years after Lister's discovery. Today, we take almost immediate adoption of scientific advance for granted. A 13-year delay in the late 19th century was actually a pretty quick adoption of this major advance. Today, we use the "aseptic technique" of surgery: rather than treating to prevent infection caused by bacteria present on instruments and wounds, we use sterilized instruments in an environment carefully designed to prevent the introduction of bacteria into surgical wounds.

121. Quoted in Harvey Cushings's magisterial 1925 "The Life of William Osler," Vol. II, 160.

122. Dungan to BuMed, date not clear but probably August 29, 1872, RG 52, Entry 7, Box 91, Letter Book 8, August 1872, 326, 325.

123. Dungan to Surgeon General James G. Palmer, September 28, 1872, RG 52, Entry 7, Box 91, Letter Book 9, 226.

124. Browne to Beale, October 29, 1876, RG 52, Entry 7, Box 116, 1876, Letter Book 10, October, 307.

125. We know this because Gihon, in a report on sewers and drains, writes in November 1887, "All the emanations from a long sewer receiving all the sewage wastes of the Hospital is vented through this rain leader, whose open mouth is on a level with the porch roof, and within a few feet of the windows of the rooms occupied by Medical Director Gihon, U.S.N. which open directly on this porch" (my underlining). Report of a Board of Examination to Shipyard Commandant Belknap, November 30, 1887, RG 52, Entry 11, Box 18, Entry 4296B.

126. Gihon to Surgeon General John Mills Browne, September 12, 1888, RG 52, General Correspondence February 1885–April 1912, Box 22, File September 21, 1888.

127. Statistical Report on the Health of the Navy, fragment found in RG 52, Entry 11, Box 23.

128. Statistical Report on the Health of the Navy, RG 52, Entry 11, Box 29, Entry 2239.

129. Browne to the Secretary of the Navy (Received October 12, 1889), RG 52, Entry 11, Box 30, File 2660.

130. Browne to Senator W.B. Allison, April 18, 1890, RG 52, Entry 11, Box 24, File 590.

131. A packet from the Secretary of the Navy received at BuMed on September 22, 1891, includes the excerpt from the "Digest of Naval Appropriations for the Fiscal Year 1892." RG 52, Entry 11, Box 43, File 1414.

132. Secretary of the Navy to BuMed, September 22, 1891, "Digest of Naval Appropriations for Fiscal Year 1892," RG 52, Entry 1415, Box 43.

133. Hubbard was born in Holden, Massachusetts. He attended Massachusetts Institute of Technology and, after a brief practice in Cleveland, moved to Washington, D.C., in 1891, where he was in the office of the supervising architect at the Treasury Department at the time these drawings were made. This must have been one of his first "government" projects.
Massachusetts Institute of Technology, "News of the Classes," *Technology Review*, 23 (1921): 627–628, https://books.google.com/books?id=hK0PAQAAIAAJ&pg=PA627&lpg=PA627&dq=ervin+s+hubbard+architect&source=bl&ots=EP7_fJf-4q&sig=dGxljeV57nTNWOZ7AQQ

Notes—Chapter Five

VdvT_Wik&hl=en&sa=X&ved=0CDMQ6AEwCGoVChMI77yg3Yq0yAIVAT6ICh1uQQgn#v=onepage&q=ervin%20s%20hubbard%20architect&f=false.

134. Browne specified that the wiring "be run beneath the plastering and floors and the ends are to project wherever there is a gas outlet so that when the fixtures are introduced, they can be connected with them." Apparently, there were no electrical codes in 1892. Nowadays, wiring must be run behind the walls and not buried in plaster.

135. All correspondence related to construction of the hospital commander's home is contained in RG 52, Records of the Bureau of Medicine and Surgery, Headquarters Records, Correspondence, 1842–1941, General Correspondence, February 1885–April 1912, Entry 11, Boxes 43, 49, 50.

136. Navy correspondence, RG 52, Entry 11, Box 48, Entry 606, Received May 25, 1892, dated May 19, 1892. Newspaper quote, http://cdnc.ucr.edu/cgi-bin/cdnc?a=d&d=SDU18920420.2.2&e=------en--20--1---txIN--------1.

137. Telegraphic communications between Navy Yard Commandant Glass and BuMed included in a packet. RG 52, Entry 11, Box 96, File 39638.

138. Commandant W.A. Kirkland to BuMed, April 7, 1898, RG 52, Entry 11, Box 97, File 39836.

139. "Navy-Yard Severely Damaged" (headline), *San Francisco Call*, April 1, 1898, 1, https://chroniclingamerica.loc.gov/lccn/sn85066387/1898-04-01/ed-1/seq-1.

140. Telegram, Navy Yard Commandant to Surgeon General Van Reypen, Entry 11, Box 96, File 39638.

141. Surgeon General to Secretary of the Navy, April 11, 1898, RG 52, Entry 11, Box 97, File 39956.

Chapter Five

1. A June 4 letter from the bureau to the commandant of the Marine Corps specified that "this Bureau [of Medicine and Surgery] will bear one third of the expense for water and electric light at the Marine Corps Barracks, during such time as the Barracks shall be occupied by the Naval Hospital" (RG 52, Entry 11, Box 100, File 41780).

2. Extracts from a Report of Inspection of the Navy Yard, Mare Island, California, September 15, 1898. RG 52, Entry 11, Box 106, File 44590.

3. Medical Director in Charge George P. Bradley to the Surgeon General, April 20, 1898, RG 52, Entry 11, Box 98, File 40309.

4. Surgeon General Van Reypen to the Honorable Joseph G. Cannon, Chairman, Committee on Appropriations, House of Representatives, April 20, 1898, RG 52, Entry 11, Box 98, File 40310.

5. Van Reypen to the Secretary of the Navy John D. Long, May 24, 1898, RG 52, Entry 11, Box 100, File 414438. This file also contains Van Reypen's correspondence with architect W.M. Poindexter confirming his engagement to create drawings for the new hospital.

6. Acting BuMed Chief (name not recorded) to Colonel Commandant of the Marine Corps, June 6, 1898, File 41780, June 6, 1898.

7. Van Reypen to Senator George C. Perkins, July 7, 1898, RG 52, Entry 11, Box 102, File 42594, dated June 28, 1898. This file also contains Senator Perkins's letter of inquiry.

8. Requisition from BuMed to Secretary of the Navy, August 26, 1898, RG 52, Entry 11, Box 104, File 43801.

9. Surgeon General's Report to the Secretary of the Navy dated October 1, 1898, RG 52, Entry 11, Box 103, 22–24.

10. Surgeon General's Report to the Secretary of the Navy dated October 1, 1898, RG 52, Entry 11, Box 103.

11. September 3, 1898, 12, http://cdnc.ucr.edu/cgi-bin/cdnc?a=d&d=SFC18980903.2.178&e=-------en--20--1--txt-txIN--------1.

12. This entire flurry of correspondence is contained in a large packet found in RG 52, Entry 11, Box 106, File 44836, earliest date is October 12, 1898.

Notes—Chapter Six

13. Golden Gate Lodge No. 1, Plasterers of San Francisco, International Union 118, to Secretary of the Navy Long, November 16, 1898, RG 52, Entry 11, Box 118, File 52628. This is a large packet of correspondence that covers minute details of the plaster problem and problems with the contractor Dahlberg's slowness in paying his bills.

14. Correspondence in RG 52, Entry 11, Box 106, File 44836, earliest date is October 12, 1898.

15. Telegram from Navy Yard Commandant M. Miller to the Surgeon General, April 3, 1900, RG 52, Entry 11, File 52628.

16. Campbell, W.T., "The Pavilion-Style Hospital of the American Civil War and Florence Nightingale," *National Museum of Civil War Medicine* (July 8, 2019), https://www.civilwarmed.org/surgeons-call/pavilionhospitals/. The pavilion hospital design is attributed to Florence Nightingale, a British statistician cum nurse who became famous for her reform of military hospital operations while overseeing the care of British soldiers during the Crimean War. Nightingale's statistical work demonstrated that the pavilion design was associated with decreased patient morbidity and mortality. She attributed this result to the superior ventilation the design permitted.

17. Memorandum for the Secretary of the Navy (Synopsis of the Annual Report of the Surgeon-General of the Navy), October 1, 1900, RG 52, Entry 11, Box 124, File 56793.

18. Civil Engineer Stanford to the Surgeon General, June 16, 1900, RG 52, Entry 11, Box 118, File 52628.

19. Note: 32 candle-power is equivalent to 44 watts in an example from Goo, B.F., "How the Line-Wires Light Lamps," *School Science and Mathematics*, 16(1) (January 1916): 12–14, http://books.google.com/books?id=gVpLAAAAMAAJ&pg=PA12&lpg=PA12&dq=32+candlepower+%3D%3F+watts&source=bl&ots=I1C8WwHYoa&sig=mfCMADipAVnyNkDU8487TfcwEPU&hl=en&ei=IQhrTPW0OIH98Ab6q8yLBA&sa=X&oi=book_result&ct=result&resnum=3&ved=0CCMQ6AEwAg#v=onepage&q&f=false. Carbon filament light bulbs, likely those used in 1900, produced less than half the light of a modern tungsten filament bulb. Based on this, it's probable that the bulbs used in the hospital each drew about 90 watts.

20. Medical Director in Charge J.A. Hawke to Commandant Miller, November 21, 1900, RG 52, Entry 11, Box 118, File 59429 (52628).

21. Medical Director in Charge George P. Bradley to Commandant Miller, July 13, 1900, ff, RG 52, Entry 11, Box 124, File 56818. The hospital flagpole seems to be an important feature. It appears frequently in this, previous, and subsequent correspondence.

22. NAVEDTRA 14295, *Hospital Corpsman Reference* (Pensacola: Naval Education and Training Professional Development and Technology Center, 2000, revised 2003, AI-2,3), http://www.navybmr.com/NAVEDTRA%2014295.html.

23. Bradley to the Bureau, November 3, 1898, RG 52, Entry 11, Box 107, File 45576.

24. Hawke to Miller (forwarded to BuMed), January 14, 1901, RG 52, Entry 11, Box 130, File 60559.

25. Passed Assistant Surgeon A.W. Dunbar to Van Reypen, April 5, 1901, RG 52, Entry 11, Box 133, File 62393.

26. Hawke to Van Reypen, March 16, 1901, RG 52, Entry 11, Box 132, File 62136.

27. Hawke to BuMed, July 14, 1902, RG 52, Entry 11, Box 146, File 70294.

Chapter Six

1. Department of State forwards a translation of a note from the Swiss minister to Washington, D.C., to Hawke, April 16, 1901, with reply to BuMed via Department of Navigation. RG 52, Entry 11, Box 133, File 62487.

2. Hawke, handwritten letter to Van

Notes—Chapter Six

Reypen (with Van Reypen's reply), September 5, 1901, RG 52, Entry 11, Box 138, File 65558.

3. Personal: Hawke to Van Reypen, November 29, 1901, RG 52, Entry 11, Box 141, File 67188.

4. Hawke to Surgeon General, December 31, 1901, and reply, RG 52, Entry 11, Box 142, File 67817.

5. Hawke to Rixey, January 28, 1902, RG 52, Entry 11, Box 143, File 68420. This file contains all correspondence related to construction of quarters for the hospital second in charge and chief surgeon.

6. Surgeon General Rixey to the Honorable George E. Foss, M.C., Chairman, Committee on Naval Affairs, House of Representatives, April 14, 1902, RG 52, Entry 11, Box 146, File 70038.

7. Surgeon General Rixey to the Honorable George E. Foss, this entire correspondence contained in April 14, 1902, RG 52, Entry 11, Box 143, File 68420.

8. Simons to BuMed, April 20, 1904, RG 52, Entry 11, Box 181, File 86718.

9. Hawke to BuMed, July 14, 1902, RG 52, Entry 11, Box 146, File 70294.

10. Medical Director Manly H. Simons to Surgeon General Presley Marion Rixey, April 23, 1903 (and replies), RG 52, Entry 11, Box 165, File 78996.

11. Medical Director Manly H. Simons to Surgeon General Presley Marion Rixey, April 23, 1903 (and replies), RG 52, Entry 11, Box 171, File 81657; Simons to Rixey, August 20, 1903, RG 52, Entry 11, Box 171, File 81657. The requisition for the bicycle has scrawled across its face in broad pencil, "not approved cancelled."

12. Simons to Rixey, May 18, 1903, RG 52, Entry 11, Box 167, File 80012.

13. Personal Simons to Rixey, November 12, 1903, RG 52, Entry 11, Box 174, File 83615.

14. Roosevelt, T.R. (May 14, 1903), Address at the Laying of the Cornerstone of the Y.M.C.A. Auxiliary Clubhouse in Vallejo, California [Speech transcript], The American Presidency Project, https://www.presidency.ucsb.edu/documents/address-the-laying-the-cornerstone-the-ymca-auxiliary-clubhouse-vallejo-california.

15. Pharmacist Stephen St. John to Medical Officer in Charge, Naval Hospital, Mare Island, California, March 16, 1904, ff, RG 52, Entry 11, Box 180, File 86190.

16. Simons to Commandant of the Navy Yard, March 10, 1904, RG 52, Entry 11, Box 180, File 86049.

17. Report of the Surgeon General of the U.S. Navy to the Secretary of the Navy, October 1, 1904 (excerpts), RG 52, Entry 11, Box 186, File 88971.

18. Simons to Rixey, June 16, 1904, ff, RG 52, Entry 11, Box 185, File 88704.

19. Surgeon General's Report to the Secretary of the Navy ("Medicine & Surgery Estimates"), September 1, 1905, RG 52, Entry 11, Box 204, File 97698.

20. Surgeon General's Report to the Secretary of the Navy 1905, RG 52, Entry 11, Box 204, File 97685.

21. Naval Hospital, Cañacao, Philippines, near Manila, was built by the Spanish but "inherited" when the United States took control of that country after the Spanish-American War. It continued to serve the Navy until January 1942, when it was bombed, then occupied by the Japanese.

22. Infected.

23. Compound fractures are broken bones where the broken end(s) extend through the skin. They are at particular risk for infection of the bone (with a real risk of failure to heal in this era before antibiotics). "Unreduced" simply means that the fractures had been left untreated and no effort made to bring the broken ends of bone back into alignment.

24. Emitting pus—that is, another way of saying "infected."

25. Until the work of Pasteur and others established the role of bacteria in causing wound infections in the 1860s and '70s, surgery was a fraught undertaking; 35 percent or more of amputation patients died of infectious complications. The notion of "laudable pus"—that is, a creamy discharge from the wound—as carrying a good prognosis versus a thin,

Notes—Chapter Six

watery (deadly) discharge was universally accepted. British surgeon Joseph Lister was the first to try to reduce the risk of infection. He did so by spraying carbolic acid (phenol), an antiseptic, into the operating room air. This led to a substantial reduction of the rate of wounds that went bad. This first attempt at infection prevention is called "Listerism" or "antiseptic technique." Lister went further, though, ultimately advocating for surgery using sterile instruments—that is, altogether preventing the introduction of bacteria into surgical wounds. This we refer to as "aseptic" technique.

26. Report of Fleet Surgeon, Asiatic Station, June 7, 1905, RG 52, Entry 11, Box 205, File 9778x, NAB.

27. Charles N. Ellinwood, MD, President Cooper Medical College to Surgeon General Rixey, November 7, 1905, RG 52, Entry 11, Box 209, File 100352. Ellinwood was fired by the board of directors in 1906 over allegations of financial misdealings, never proven. He was a prominent San Francisco physician, said to have been director of the San Francisco Marine (Public Health) Hospital at one time.

28. F.F. Shook, Asst. Surgeon to BuMed, April 17, 1906, ff, RG 52, Records of the Bureau of Medicine and Surgery, Headquarters Records, Medical Journals and Reports on Patients, Navy Medical Logs and Reports 1870–1941; Mare Island 1905–1906 NARS A-1 Box 038 Entry 22A, Vol. [unlabeled] of 2.

29. Telegram, B.H. McCalla to the Bureau of Navigation, April 18, 1906, forwarded to the Bureau of Medicine and Surgery, April 23, 1906, ff, RG 52, Entry 11, Box 223, File 103962.

30. Simons to BuMed, June 1, 1906, RG 52, Entry 11, Box 224, File 104628.

31. BuMed to Hospital Commanding Officer, July 9, 1906, RG 52, Entry 11, Box 227, File 105680.

32. Persons to Bureau, March 30, 1907, ff, RG 52, Entry 11, Box 241, File 111470.

33. Persons to BuMed in response to a circular letter requesting a list of repairs made in 1907, and recommended future work, "Report of Improvements and Repairs Made at the Naval Hospital, Mare Island, Cal., during the fiscal year, 1906–1907, June 5, 1907," RG 52, Entry 11, Box 243, File 112062.

34. Hospital Commander to BuMed, October 22, 1906, ff, RG 52, Entry 11, Box 231, File 107806.

35. Rest, recreation, exercise, a wholesome diet.

36. Chest X-ray is a key step in diagnosing tuberculosis, which usually affects the lungs. The new "Standard Navy X-Ray Outfit" played an essential role here.

37. Persons to BuMed, January 7, 1907, Report on the Cases of Pulmonary Tuberculosis Treated in the Camp at the Naval Hospital, Mare Island, Calif, 1906, RG 52, Entry 11, Box 236, File 110282.

38. Including the hospital ship USS *Relief*.

39. Personal: Rixey to Persons, February 6, 1908, RG 52, Entry 11, Box 257.

40. Persons to the Surgeon General, September 26, 1908, RG 52, Entry 11, Box 267, File 115965.

41. Annual Report of the Surgeon General, U.S. Navy to the Secretary of the Navy for the Fiscal Year 1909 (1909), U.S. Government Printing Office, pp. 122–123, https://books.google.com/books?id=b6yCesjD0EoC&pg=RA3-PA159&lpg=RA3-PA159&dq=navy+surgeon+general%27s+report+1908&source=bl&ots=vAmHsqmi4w&sig=ACfU3U0GROFJQJ2hsCC3ksOBsv323_X_Dw&hl=en&sa=X&ved=2ahUKEwj4g5-p5Y7-AhXFOn0KHSKhDl44KBDoAXoECAQQAw#v=onepage&q=navy%20surgeon%20general's%20report%201908&f=false.

42. Hospital Commander to BuMed, July 1, 1908, RG 52, Entry 11, Box 263, File 115285.

43. Persons to Rixey, February 17, 1909, RG 52, Entry 11, Box 272, File 116423.

44. Assistant Surgeon General William Clarence Braisted to Simons, December 2, 1909, ff, RG 52, Entry 11, Box 291, File 118860.

Notes—Chapter Seven

45. Simons to Surgeon General Charles F. Stokes, March 26, 1910, Surgeon General's Report to the Secretary of the Navy, RG 52, Entry 11, Box 291, File 118860.

46. BuMed Circular Letter to Naval Hospitals Annapolis, Mare Island, Cañacao, Las Animas, Norfolk, Yokohama, January 22, 1909, RG 52, Entry 11, Box 275, File 116628.

47. Correspondence between BuMed and the Secretary of the Navy about Nurse Corps housing; Mare Island appears on the approval list, but no correspondence specific to Mare Island appears in this file. RG 52, Entry 11, Box 277, File 116771.

48. Correspondence between BuMed and the Secretary of the Navy, RG 52, Entry 11, Box 227, File 117751 (contained in packet 105680).

49. Simons to Stokes, February 17, 1910, RG 52, Entry 11, Box 297, File 119465.

50. This was entered as a file space filler, dated July 5, 1910, with a hand-entered statement regarding Miss Anna Turner, dated June 6, 1910, RG 52, Entry 11, Box 303, File 120579 (subordinated to 115738).

51. Simons to Stokes, September 22, 1910, RG 52, Entry 11, Box 307, File 121191.

52. Simons to Rixey, February 1910, RG 52, Entry 11, Box 227, File 117751.

53. Simons to Rixey, February 1910, RG 52, Entry 11, Box 227, File 119401.

54. Simons to the Surgeon General, December 10, 1910, RG 52, Entry 11, Box 310, Files 121694 and 122058.

55. Annual Report of the Surgeon General (Charles F. Stokes) to the Secretary of the Navy, June 21, 1911, RG 52, Entry 11, Box 320, File 123003.

56. Phillips A. Lovering to BuMed, August 3, 1911, RG 52, Entry 11, Box 322, File 123299.

57. Lovering to the Surgeon General, August 3, 1911, RG 52, Entry 11, Box 322, Files 123299 and 123410.

58. Secretary of the Navy General Order 148, Liability Act, January 31, 1912, RG 52, Entry 11, Box 329, File 124448.

59. For instance, Lovering admitted Ah Loy, civilian cook, "as with enteritis" to hospital in December 1911, based on (in pencil) "Standing authority for adm of Hosp. employees (civ) as sup[ernumaries]. Without ref of ea[ch] case to Bur[eau]." Entry 11, Box 327, File 124179.

60. Gates to Surgeon General, June 18, 1913, RG 52, Entry 11, Box 327, File 124179.

61. Medical Director Manly F. Gates to Surgeon General Braisted, February 20, 1914, RG 52, Records of the Bureau of Medicine and Surgery, Headquarters Records Correspondence, 1842–1941, General Correspondence March 1912–December 1925, Entry 12, Box 455, File 126294-12 Mare Island.

62. Gates to BuMed, January 18, 1915, RG 52, Entry 12, Box 487, File 126885-12 Mare Island.

63. Annual Report of the Surgeon General, U.S. Navy, Chief of the Bureau of Medicine and Surgery, to the Secretary of the Navy for the Fiscal Year 1916 (1916) U.S. Government Printing Office, 26, https://www.google.com/books/edition/Annual_Report_of_the_Surgeon_General_U_S/cAR_TxgNk9IC?hl=en&gbpv=1.

Chapter Seven

1. Navy Secretary Josephus Daniels, Annual Reports of the Navy Department for the Fiscal Year 1917, Annual Report of the Secretary of the Navy (1918) U.S. Government Printing Office (p. 1), https://babel.hathitrust.org/cgi/pt?id=njp.32101043274214&view=1up&seq=13&q1=798.

2. Navy Secretary Josephus Daniels, Annual Reports of the Navy Department for the Fiscal Year 1917, Annual Report of the Secretary of the Navy (1918), 3.

3. Navy Secretary Josephus Daniels, Annual Reports of the Navy Department for the Fiscal Year 1917, Annual Report of the Secretary of the Navy (1918), 60.

Notes—Chapter Seven

4. And as is, was, and likely ever shall be, "the excessive cost of labor and materials for the emergency hospital buildings at the Naval Hospital Reservation, Mare Island ... have so increased the cost of the work." Chief of the Bureau of Yards and Docks to the Chief of the Bureau of Medicine and Surgery, October 5, 1917, Entry 12, Box 551, File 128780 Mare Island.

5. Metropolitan Transportation Commission—Association of Bay Area Governments, *Bay Area Census*, City of Vallejo, Decennial Census Data for the Years 1880–1940, http://www.bayareacensus.ca.gov/cities/Vallejo50.htm#1940.

6. Secretary of the Navy's 1917 Annual Report, 63.

7. The Bureau of Yards and Docks was responsible for arranging most construction on Navy yards and bases. Its stream of funding was different from that of the Bureau of Medicine and Surgery, the construction funding for which was largely used for maintenance and emergency construction needs.

8. NARA Records of the Bureau of Medicine and Surgery, source cited before, Entry 12, Box 551, File 128780-15 Mare Island.

9. Farenholt to Braisted, March 24, 1918, RG 52, Entry 12, Box 578, File 130107 D-12 Mare Island 1918. By this time, hospital commanders were sending weekly "semi-official" letters of report to the Surgeon General.

10. Farenholt to Braisted, May 11, 1918.

11. Armed Forces Institute of Pathology (1997), *The AFIP Letter* 155(2), cited in Snyder, Thomas L., "The Great Flu Crisis at Mare Island Navy Yard, and Vallejo, California," *Navy Medicine*, 94(5) (2003): 25–29.

12. A terrific reconstruction of the 1918 flu and its effects on the body can be found in Barbara Jester, T. Uyeki, D. Jernigan, and T. Tumpey, "Historical and Clinical Aspects of the 1918 H1N1 Pandemic in the United States," *Virology*, 527 (2019): 32–37, https://www.sciencedirect.com/science/article/pii/S0042682218303313?via%3Dihub.

13. Nelson, J. L., "Influenza Epidemic, Mare Island, Cal; Special Report On" to the Navy Bureau of Medicine and Surgery (1919): (page 4, paragraph 5), from the collection of the Vallejo Naval and Historical Museum.

14. Farenholt's weekly "semi-official" letters are all contained in RG 52, Entry 12, Box 578, File 130107 D-12 Mare Island 1918.

15. "Semi-official" letters, RG 52, Entry 12, Box 578, File 130107 D-12 Mare Island 1918.

16. Snyder (2003).

17. Farenholt to Surgeon General, December 18, 1918, RG 52, Entry 12, Box 578, File 130107. This file contains Farenholt's semi-official letters to the bureau from February 4 to December 28, 1918.

18. Farenholt to BuMed, semi-official letter, January 4, 1919, RG 52, Box 578, File 13017 D-12 Mare Island 1919, 11–54. Patients who survived the cytokine storm-related lung inflammation often fell victim to "secondary" bacterial lung infections. The pneumococcus bacterium is a common cause of pneumonia even today, and today we can receive immunizations against the infection in the form of "Pneumovax." In Miss Caterline's case, the bacteria had spread to her blood stream—"septicemia." There were no antibiotics in those days.

19. The Mare Island Naval Cemetery received its first burial soon after establishment of the Navy Yard in 1854. It was administered by the naval hospital (on the theory that "if you can't cure them, you'll still have to take care of them"). About 400 sailors, including three Congressional Medal of Honor awardees, and family members are buried there. When the Navy Yard closed in 1996, cemetery ownership was ceded to the city of Vallejo. The city's bankruptcy and general apathy led to a serious decline of the cemetery's status. Finally, in 2020, legislation sponsored by Congressman Mike Thompson and Senator Dianne Feinstein directed that the cemetery be taken

Notes—Chapter Eight

over by the Department of Veterans Affairs. The official transfer of ownership occurred in November 2023.

20. Farenholt, semi-official letter, January 10, 1919, RG 52, Entry 12, Box 578, File 130107 D-12 Mare Island 1919, 11–54.

Chapter Eight

1. Farenholt, January 17, 1919, RG 52, Entry 12, Box 578, File 130107 D-12 Mare Island 1919, 11–54.

2. Annual Report of the Surgeon General, U.S. Navy to the Secretary of the Navy for the Fiscal Year 1919 (1919), U.S. Government Printing Office (p. 5), https://www.google.com/books/edition/Annual_report_of_the_Surgeon_General_U_S/zV4xe7NLDfsC?hl=en&gbpv=1&dq=annual+report+of+the+Surgeon+General+of+the+Navy+fiscal+year+1919&pg=PA122&printsec=frontcover.

3. Farenholt, January 24, RG 52, Entry 12, Box 578, File 130107 D-12 Mare Island 1919, 11–54.

4. This number is somewhat deceiving. A list from November 28, 1919, reports total patients of 834 but just 320 "bed patients." Presumably, the 514 others were ambulatory, requiring a bed, a roof, three square meals a day and minimal nursing care. Nevertheless, the men in those ambulatory facilities need bedding changes, showers and baths and food preparation.

5. The Bureau of War Risk Insurance was established by Congress in 1914, initially to indemnify commercial shipping from loss due to acts of war. An amendment to the act, passed in October 1917, added sections that provided for servicemember life insurance (recall that most commercial life insurance policies specifically exclude losses due to "acts of war or insurrection"), and more pertinent to our narrative, "the injured person shall be furnished by the United States such reasonable governmental medical, surgical, and hospital services and with such supplies, including artificial limbs, trusses, and similar appliances, as the director may determine to be useful and reasonably necessary." "Hospital Provision for Disabled War Veterans—An American Report," *British Medical Journal*, 3251 (1923): 685–686, https://www.ncbi.nlm.nih.gov/pmc/articles/PMC2316102/pdf/brmedj06262-0021b.pdf.

6. Farenholt, August 31, 1919.

7. Braisted to the Chief of Naval Operations Admiral Robert E. Coontz, April 17, 1920, RG 52, Entry 12, Box 628, File 132610 D-12 Mare Island Hospital.

8. Farenholt semi-official letter to BuMed, May 31, 1920, RG 52, Entry 12, Box 578, File D-12 Mare Island 1920 130307.

9. Farenholt to BuMed, April 29, 1920, RG 52, Entry 12, Box 578, File 130107 D-12 Mare Island 1919, 11–54.

10. Farenholt to BuMed, June 30, 1919, RG 52, Entry 12, Box 578, File 130107 D-12 Mare Island, 64–126.

11. Report of Inspection, U.S. Naval Hospital, Mare Island, California, July 9th and 10th, 1919. A.M.D. McCormick, Rear Admiral, Medical Corps, U.S. Navy, Inspecting Officer. Summary of Inspection Report, Suggested Changes or Improvements. RG 52, Entry 12, Box 616, File 132578 D-12, Mare Island 1.

12. Stitt to the Bureau of Yards and Docks, July 26, 1922, RG 52, Entry 12, Box 645, File 132687-D12 Mare Island Hospital.

13. Stitt to Secretary of the Navy Edwin Denby, July 11, 1923, RG 52, Entry 12, Box 647, File 132690 D-0 1923 General, NAB.

14. First Indorsement [sic] from the Chief of the Bureau of Yards and Docks to the Secretary of the Navy, July 12, 1923, RG 52, Entry 12, Box 647, File 132690 D-0 1923 General, NAB.

15. Braisted to the Bureau of Yards and Docks, January 28, 1919, RG 52, Entry 12, Box 622, File 132600-D12 (1919).

16. Stitt to Commandant, Navy Yard, May 10, 1922, RG 52, Entry 12, Box 645, File 132687-D12 (1922).

17. The Veterans' Bureau was the precursor to today's Department of Veterans Affairs.

18. Dunbar to Captain C.P. Kindleberger, May 14, 1925, RG 52, Entry 12, Box 660, File 132692-D12 (1925).

19. Kindleberger to Surgeon General, June 21, 1926, RG 52, Entry 15a, Box 123, Files NH15 L11-1 to S38-1 1926–1939, NAB.

20. "Award Contract to Build Navy Hospital for Mare Island," *San Pedro News [Daily] Pilot*, 1926, 1. California Digital Newspaper Collection: 13(150), https://cdnc.ucr.edu/?a=d&d=SPNP19260324.2.35&e=-------en--20--1--txt-txIN--------.

21. Kindleberger to Surgeon General, April 20, 1927, ff, RG 52, Entry 15A, Box 123, File NH 15 / N4-1 to NH 15 / N 9 (1926–1941).

22. Kindleberger to Surgeon General, January 12, 1928, RG 52, Entry 15A, Box 123, File NH 15 / N 13-1 to NH 15 / S 38-1.

Chapter Nine

1. Physical copies of the *Times-Herald* are retained in the archives of the Vallejo Naval and Historical Museum, 734 Marin Street, Vallejo, California 94590.

2. Hospital Commander J.A. Murphy to Surgeon General Admiral C.E. Riggs, January 30, 1931, ff, RG 52, Entry 15A, Box 122, File NH15 (A1-1 to L9-3), 1936–1941, NAB.

3. May 2015. The renovation was largely paid for by the Jelly Belly candy company.

4. KTAB got its call letters from its original home, the Tenth Avenue Baptist Church in Oakland. Many churches opened radio stations in the late 1920s and early 1930s with the intention of broadcasting services on Sundays. The temptation for "commercial" operations was strong, however, and many stations, including KTAB, continued broadcasting, though at reduced power, on weekdays. In 1933, KTAB moved its main studios to San Francisco and shortly thereafter changed its call letters to KSFO. This station remains a Bay Area broadcast powerhouse to this day. Bay Area Radio Museum, Bay Area Radio Hall of Fame, "Timeline KSFO," https://bayarearadio.org/history-index/timeline_ksfo.

5. *Times Herald*, March 4, 1933.

6. *Times Herald*, June 27, 1934.

7. Grayson, a Navy physician, had been Woodrow Wilson's personal physician and played a notorious role in covering up Wilson's severe disability from a stroke suffered while in office.

8. Furer, J.A., *Administration of the Navy Department in World War II*, U.S. Government Printing Office. Chapter XII, Bureau of Medicine and Surgery, 487, https://www.ibiblio.org/hyperwar/USN/Admin-Hist/USN-Admin/USN-Admin-12.html.

9. Guthrie, Chester L. (ed.), *The United States Naval Medical Department at War—1941–1945*. (Unpublished, 1946); *The United States Navy Medical Department Administrative History, Volume I*, Administrative History Section, Administrative Section, Bureau of Medicine and Surgery, Navy Department. Chapters I–VI. Operations Narrative. Introduction, 1, https://digirepo.nlm.nih.gov/ext/dw/14321920RX1/PDF/14321920RX1.pdf.

Chapter Ten

1. Avery, B. F. (ed.), *The History of the Medical Department of the United States Navy in World War II Volume 1* (Washington, DC: U.S. Government Printing Office), Chapter 1.

2. This packet of correspondence is found in RG 52, Entry 15A, Box 122, File NH15 (A1-1 to L-93) (1936–1941).

3. This correspondence is also in RG 52, Entry 15A, Box 122, File NH15 (A1-1 to L9-3).

4. "Medicine: Burns at Mare Island," *Time*, November 16, 1942, https://con

Notes—Chapter Ten

tent.time.com/time/subscriber/article/0,33009,932877-1,00.html.

5. The Navy medical department's prewar numbers stood at about 860 doctors. By war's end, more than 14,000 served wounded and sick sailors and Marines.

6. Captain A.L. Clifton (Commanding Officer) to Luther Sheldon at BuMed, January 12, 1942, RG 52, Entry 15B, Box 104, File NH15/A1-1, National Archives, College Park, Maryland (hereafter NACP).

7. Holman, E., "Gunshot Wounds of the Heart: Subsequent Removal of Foreign Bodies. Two Case Reports," *U.S. Navy Medical Bulletin*, 40(951) (1942). Holman reports operating "with trepidation for fear of massive bleeding" (from the heart itself!). Remember, surgeons and anesthesiologists didn't have sophisticated equipment like heart-lung machines or modern drugs and techniques for major cardiac surgery in that time. Fortunately, the patients were otherwise healthy young men.

8. From Holman's Service Record, a copy of which the author obtained from the Navy Records Section of the National Archives in St. Louis, Missouri.

9. Reed's Inspection Report to BuMed, February 7, 1942, RG 52, Entry 15B, Box 104, Folder NH15/A1-1 to NH16/L5-3, File NH15/a10-2 TO nh15/l8-2.

10. By now, it must be clear that a good many of these patients weren't very ill or were sufficiently recovered from surgery or illness so as not to require much more than a bed, a roof and three square meals a day while they awaited reassignment back to the forces or discharge from the service.

11. Reed's Inspection Report to BuMed, August 21, 1943, RG 52, Entry 15A, Box 104, File NH15/A10-2 to L8-2.

12. The Waves (Women Accepted for Volunteer Emergency Service) program was signed into law by Franklin D. Roosevelt on July 30, 1942, and was intended to free up male personnel for sea and combat duty. Officer Waves served as cryptographers, communications specialists, translators, meteorologists and engineers. Enlisted Waves became medical technicians ("Corps Waves"), radio operators, yeomen (secretaries), supply technicians and cooks.

13. Captain John P. Owen (Hospital Commander) personal to McIntire, November 25, 1942, RG 52, Entry 15B, Box 104, Folder NH15/A1-1 to NH16/L5-3, File NH15/L9-3. Captain Clifton went on to command the Naval Convalescent Hospital in Sun Valley, Idaho. He returned to Mare Island in September 1944 for surgical repair of a broken elbow. He died of a heart attack in Sun Valley five months later.

14. Owen to BuMed, September 15, 1943, RG 52, Entry 15B, Box 104, NH15/A1-1 to NH16/L5-3, File NH15/A1-1.

15. Owen personal to McIntire, September 14, 1943.

16. Greene, R.S., *Breaking Point—The Ironic Evolution of Psychiatry in World War II* (New York: Fordham University Press, 2023). Greene's history of pre- and wartime psychiatry is comprehensive. The prewar history of the plans for screening is contained in pages 1–35.

17. Holman and Reed to BuMed, a string of correspondence from January April 18, 1940, to February 3, 1941, in RG 52, Entry 15A, Box 122, File NH15 (A1-1 to L9-3), 1936–1941.

18. Reed's Inspection Report to BuMed, February 7, 1942, RG 52, Entry Box 104 (NH15/A1-1 to NH16/L5-3), File NH15/A10-2 to NH15/L8-2.

19. Reed's Inspection Report to BuMed, May 29, 1942.

20. St. Elizabeth's Hospital in Washington, D.C., opened in 1855 as the first federal hospital for the care of the mentally ill. During World War II, the Navy sent officers suffering from psychoses to St. Elizabeth's.

21. Guthrie, 97–100. The Navy had a contract with the Public Health Service (PHS) for care of psychotic patients. The PHS hospital in Fort Worth was the agreed site for this care. By the end of 1944, 11 Navy physicians and 138 corpsmen assisted in the care of Navy patients

Notes—Chapter Ten

at the hospital alongside 136 PHS personnel. The hospital cared for more than 4,000 Navy and Marine Corps psychotic patients during the war. https://digirepo.nlm.nih.gov/ext/dw/14321920RX1/PDF/14321920RX1.pdf.

22. Clifton to BuMed, April 20, 1942, RG 52, Entry 15B, Box 104 (NH15/A101 to NH16/L5-3), File NH/15/L16-8 to NH15/S85.

23. Correspondence in RG 52, Entry 15B, Box 118, Folder NH70-7-0000015-3 to NH70-9—A4-2, NACP. These are Bureau of Personnel files but located in BuMed folders.

24. The inn may have been BuMed's foster child, however. A letter to a citizen inquiring about massage therapy treatments for personnel staying at the inn had penciled in, "19 Apr '43—Secnav (Secretary of the Navy) to Com[mander] Serv[ice] Force, Pacific Flt, Subordinate Command—Nav[al] Rest Center, Sonoma Mission Inn." This suggests that the inn was really not in the BuMed chain of command.

25. Furer.

26. And others: sexual assault victims represent the largest single group of people suffering PTSD.

27. Toffelmier was an Oakland, California, orthopedist and a Navy Reservist. After the war, he returned to his Oakland practice and enjoyed a distinguished career that included tours as a rehabilitation expert on state and national panels.

28. During World War II, the Mare Island Navy Yard *Grapevine* bore the motto, "Mare Island Ships Are Fighting Everywhere." The paper, started in 1941 as a monthly, became a weekly, published every Friday, by January 1943. It remained in publication until the Navy Yard closed in 1996.

29. All patients from the Pacific theater of war undergoing amputations were to be sent to Mare Island as soon as possible so proper preparation of their limbs for prosthetic fitting could be performed. The Philadelphia naval hospital received the same designation for the European theater of war.

30. An inspection report from the 12th Naval District Medical Officer in October 1949 detailed the missions of the Brace Shop, aka West Coast Amputation Center, as "a. Conduct of research in development of artificial appliances under auspices of the National Research Council, Committee on Artificial Limbs, in conjunction with the University of California as their Veterans' Administration project on artificial limbs; b. Conduct classes in training, when arranged, for civilian limb fitters; c. Conduct training school in the manufacture of orthopedic appliances for hospital corps personnel; d. Manufacture artificial limbs and appliances for Veterans' Administration in-patients and train patients in their use; e. Furnish artificial limbs for Guamian [sic] Amputees, war casualties and others; f. Furnish automobile driving instruction and training of amputees." 12th Naval District Medical Officer Inspection Report to BuMed, October 10, 1949, RG 52, Records of the Bureau of Medicine and Surgery, General Correspondence, 1947–1951, Entry 15C, Box 111, File NH15/A10-3.

31. Early researcher and engineer Howard T. Eberhart, himself an amputee (due to a crush injury suffered while doing research on B-29 landing gear at Hamilton Field, California), along with University of California, San Francisco orthopedist Dr. Verne T. Inman, sought the Mare Island device in late 1945. Although it was the best at the time, its imperfections led Eberhart and Inman to embark on their pioneering biomechanical research. "Progress in Prosthetics" (1962) Office of Vocational Rehabilitation, U.S. Department of Health, Education, and Welfare, Washington, DC, www.oandplibrary.org/assets/pdf/ProgressInProsthetics.pdf.

32. McIntire to Holman, December 5, 1941, RG52, Entry 15A, Box 122, File NH 15 (A1-1 to L9-3) 1936–1941, NAB.

33. The average hospital stay for today's obstetric cases is about three days.

34. Owen to McIntire, September

Notes—Chapter Eleven

15, 1943, RG 52, Entry 15B, Box 104, Folder NH15/1-1 to NH16/L5-3, File NH15/A1-1, NACP.

35. In the early 2000s, whenever I led people on tours of the hospital grounds, I would inevitably be asked, "I was born at Mare Island; can you show me where?" That third-floor area no longer exists, having been demolished some time after the war. In the late 1990s, I'm told, there were still occasional informal BAMI—Born at Mare Island—meetings.

Chapter Eleven

1. Captain Wendell H. Perry to RADM Clifford A Swanson (Surgeon General), October 20, 1948, RG 52, Entry 15C, Box 111, File NH15/A1-1.

2. Chief, Procurement Division, Supply Service, Veterans Administration to Surgeon General, August 24, 1949, forwarded to CO Mare Island Hospital, August 29, 1949, RG 52, Entry 15C, Box 111, File NH15/A1-1.

3. Swanson to Secretary of the Navy Francis P. Matthews, February 1, 1950, RG 52, Entry 15C, Box 111, File NH15/A1-1.

4. Captain Bartholemew Hogan to Swanson, March 7, 1950, RG 52, Entry 15C, Box 112, NH15/L5-3 to NH16/A1-1, File NH15/M.

5. Hogan ("Dear Cliff") to Surgeon General Swanson, February 6, 1950, RG 52, Entry 15C, Box 111, File NH15/A1-1.

6. Captain O.B. Morrison (BuMed) to Hogan, April 26, 1950, RG 52, Entry 15C, Box 111, File NH15/A1-1.

7. Hogan was a larger-than-life figure in Vallejo civic life. His home was the only hospital in the city during the 1918 flu pandemic. He had an active practice of medicine for many years. His lobbying efforts on behalf of the Navy Yard earned him the esteem of the city of Vallejo. A public school was named for him in 1955. Originally a high school, it's now Hogan Middle School.

8. Camp Stonemen was a 2.8 million–acre Army Replacement and Reclassification and Prisoner of War Camp located near Pittsburg, California. It sprang into existence after the Pearl Harbor attack on the United States and closed after the Korean War in 1954. It's said that 1.5 million soldiers passed through its gates on the way to the wars in the Pacific.

9. This section is based on correspondence contained in files found at the National Archives facility in College Park, Maryland, as RG 52, Records of the Bureau of Medicine and Surgery, Headquarter Records, Correspondence, 1842–1951, General Correspondence, 1947–1951, Entry 15C, Boxes 1, 12, 111, 112.

10. Surgeon General H. Lamont Pugh to Hospital Commander H.V. Packard, July 7, 1952, RG 52, Entry 15C, Box 389, File NH15/A23.

11. Pugh to Packard.

12. This alludes to a "purple suit" military medical establishment. Personnel of all three services—Army, Air Force and Navy—would serve in a unified medical service, the "purple suit" being the notional color of uniform if the colors of all the services were mixed together. The idea wasn't new. General Dwight D. Eisenhower, soon after World War II ended, wrote, "After giving careful consideration to the problem of providing medical service for the Armed Forces, I have reached a conclusion that there is but one real solution, the establishment of one single, integrated medical service.... To my mind it is absolutely silly to have individual service medical systems" (quoted by Colonel Bruce W. McVeigh, Army Medical Corps, in a paper written while he was a Naval War College student, now inaccessible). Upon my release from active Navy service in 1973, I received a survey inquiring about my opinion regarding "purple suit medicine." "It would never fly with sailors," I wrote. "There's no way they would tolerate being cared for by an Army doctor." In October 2013, the Defense Health Agency was stood up. While Navy doctors still wear Navy uniforms and Air Force nurses still wear Air Force uniforms, much of

Notes—Chapter Eleven

the military medical establishment has been unified. Supply, for instance, is now under one agency. The training of Navy corpsmen and Army medics is done at one center, at Joint Base San Antonio. Even the former National Naval Medical Center in Bethesda, Maryland, designed and dedicated by Franklin D. Roosevelt, is now the Walter Reed Military Medical Center. An Army brigadier general has authority over the medical center as of this writing.

13. Tisdale to Captain Clarence Brown, August 9, 1953, RG 52, Entry 1004A, Bureau of Medicine and Surgery Administrative Division General Correspondence 1952–1971, Box 389, NH14/A23 through NH14/L10-5 to NH15/A23, January 1952–May 1952, File NH15/A1-1 December 1951–December 1955.

14. Brown to Tisdale (telegram), August 15, 1953, RG 52, Entry 1004A, Bureau of Medicine and Surgery Administrative Division General Correspondence 1952–1971, Box 389, NH14/A23 through NH14/L10-5 to NH15/A23, January 1952–May 1952, File NH15/A1-1 December 1951–December 1955.

15. Assistant Secretary of the Navy for Air to Assistant Secretary of the Navy (Health and Medical), August 4, 1954, RG 52, Entry 1004A, Bureau of Medicine and Surgery Administrative Division General Correspondence 1952–1971, Box 389, NH14/A23 through NH14/L10-5 to NH15/A23, January 1952–May 1952, File NH15/A1-1 December 1951–December 1955.

16. SECNAV Notice 5450, February 17, 1956, RG 52, Entry 1004(A), Box 606, General Correspondence 1952–1971, NH14/LL to NH15/P16/1, File NH15/A3 through NH15/A6-6.

17. Perkins (Hospital Commander) to Hogan, October 11, 1956, RG 52, Entry 1004(A), Box 606, NH14/LL to NH15/P16-1, Folder NH15/A8-3 through NH15/A12.

18. Bradley to Baldwin, April 8, 1957, RG 52, Entry 1004(A), NH13/N4-1 to NH15/A15, Box 720, Entry No. 65A4397, Folder NH15/A1-1 through NH15/A3-1.

19. Bradley to Baldwin, April 8, 1957.

20. Berry to Baldwin, July 9, 1957, RG 52, Entry 1004(A), NH13/N4-1 to NH15/A15, Box 720, Entry No. 65A4397, Folder NH15/A4-2.

21. Stone to Knowland, July 9, 1957, RG 52, Entry 1004(A), NH13/N4-1 to NH15/A15, Box 720, Entry No. 65A4397, Folder NH15/A4-2.

22. Luther Gibson telegram to Surgeon General Hogan, July 17, 1957, RG 52, Entry 1004(A), NH13/N4-1 to NH15/A15, Box 720, Entry No. 65A4397, Folder NH15/A4-2.

23. Burke to Kuchel, August 12, 1957, RG 52, Entry 1004(A), NH13/N4-1 to NH15/A15, Box 720, Entry No. 65A4397, Folder NH15/A4-2.

Bibliography

Primary Sources

Government Archives
National Archives Building, Washington, D.C., Records of
    U.S. Navy Bureau of Medicine and Surgery, Record Group 52
    U.S. Navy Bureau of Yards and Docks, Record Group 71
National Archives at College Park, Maryland, Records of
    U.S. Navy Bureau of Medicine and Surgery, Record Group 52
National Archives and Records Administration—Pacific Region (San Francisco), Records of
    U.S. Navy Bureau of Yards and Dock, Record Group 181

Newspapers
Alta California
Grapevine/The Mare Island *Grapevine*
San Francisco Call
Vallejo Evening Chronicle
Vallejo Times-Herald

Official Reports and Histories
Annual Report of the Secretary of the Navy for the Fiscal Year 1917, U.S. Government Printing Office, 1918.
Annual Report of the Surgeon General of the U.S. Navy to the Secretary of the Navy for the Fiscal Year 1919, U.S. Government Printing Office, 1919.
Avery, B.F., ed., *The History of the Medical Department of the United States Navy in World War II* (NAVMED P-5031) (Washington, D.C.: U.S. Government Printing Office, 1953).
Furer, J.A., *Administration of the Navy Department in World War II* (Washington, D.C.: U.S. Government Printing Office, 1959).
Guthrie, C.L., ed., *The United States Navy Medical Department Administrative History—1941–1945*, 1946. (Unpublished)
Hamersly, L.R., *The Records of Living Officers of the U.S. Navy and Marine Corps* (New York: J. B. Lippincott, 1878).
Johnson, A., *Message from the President of the United States to the Two Houses of Congress at the Commencement of the Third Session of the Fortieth Congress with the Reports of the Heads of Departments and Selections from Accompanying Documents.* U.S. Government Printing Office, 1869. https://books.google.com/books?id=gMxDMQEp8YMC&printsec=frontcover&source=gbs_ge_summary_r&cad=0#v=onepage&q&f=false.

Bibliography

Kendrick, D.B., *Blood Program in World War II* (Washington, D.C.: U.S. Government Printing Office, 1964).

Nelson, J.L., *Influenza Epidemic, Mare Island, Cal; Special Report On.* (Unpublished). The Vallejo Naval and Historical Museum, Vallejo, California, 1919.

Speech

Roosevelt, T.R., Address of President Roosevelt at the Laying of the Corner Stone of the Y.M.C.A. Auxiliary [sic] Club House, Vallejo, California, May 14, 1903.

Journal/Periodical Articles

Holman, E., Lt. Cmdr., M.C., U.S.N.R., "Gunshot Wounds of the Heart: Subsequent Removal of Foreign Bodies. Two Case Reports," *U.S. Nav. M. Bull.* 40 (1942): 951–954.

"Medicine: Burns at Mare Island," *Time*, November 16, 1942. https://content.time.com/time/subscriber/article/0,33009,932877-1,00.html.

Secondary Sources

Books

The American Heritage Dictionary of the English Language (4th Edition) (Boston: Houghton Mifflin, 2000).

Cormack, Joseph M., *The Legal Tender Cases—A Drama of American Legal and Financial History* (Williamsburg, VA: William and Mary Faculty Publications, 1929). https://scholarship.law.wm.edu/facpubs/1497.

Cutler, D.W., and Cutler, T.J., eds., *Dictionary of Naval Abbreviations* (Sixth Edition). (Annapolis: United States Naval Institute Press, 2005).

Ellison, Joseph, *California and the Nation 1850–1869* (Boston: Da Capo, 1969). This is a reprint of the original work which appeared as volume XVI of *Publications in History* (Berkeley: University of California Press, 1927).

Greene, R.S., *Breaking Point—The Ironic Evolution of Psychiatry in World War II* (New York: Fordham University Press, 2023).

Langley, H.D., *A History of Medicine in the Early U.S. Navy* (Baltimore: Johns Hopkins University Press, 1995).

Lott, Arnold S., *A Long Line of Ships: Mare Island's Century of Naval Activity in California* (Annapolis: United States Naval Institute Press, 1954).

NAVEDTRA 14295, *Hospital Corpsman Reference* (Pensacola: Naval Education and Training Professional Development and Technology Center, 2000, revised 2003). http://www.navybmr.com/NAVEDTRA%2014295.html.

Parker, Harry, ed., *Kidder-Parker Architects' and Builders' Handbook (18th Edition)* (Hoboken: Wiley, 1942).

Risse, G.B., *Mending Bodies, Saving Souls: A History of Hospitals* (Oxford: Oxford University Press, 1999).

Wylie, W.G., *Hospitals: Their History, Organization and Construction* (Orlando: Appleton, 1877).

Journal Articles

The Armed Forces Institute of Pathology Letter 155, no. 2 (1997).

Campbell, W.T., "The Pavilion-Style Hospital of the American Civil War and Florence

Bibliography

Nightingale," *National Museum of Civil War Medicine*, July 8, 2019. https://www.civilwarmed.org/surgeons-call/pavilionhospitals/.

Goo, B.F., "How the Line-Wires Light Lamps," *School Science and Mathematics* 16, no. 1 (1916). http://books.google.com/books?id=gVpLAAAAMAAJ&pg=PA1 2&lpg=PA12&dq=32+candlepower+%3D%3D+%3F+watts&source=bl&ots=I 1C8WwHYoa&sig=mfCMADipAVnyNkDU8487TfcwEPU&hl=en&ei=IQhrT PW0OIH98Ab6q8yLBA&sa=X&oi=book_result&ct=result&resnum=3&ved=0CCM Q6AEwAg#v=onepage&q&f=false.

Mann, W.L., "The Origin and Early Development of Naval Medicine," *United States Naval Institute Proceedings* 55, no. 319 (1929): 772ff. https://www.usni.org/magazines/proceedings/1929/september/origin-arid-early-development-naval-medicine.

Retief, F., and Cilliers, L.P., "The Influence of Christianity on Medicine from Graeco-Roman Times up to the Renaissance," *Acta Theologica* 26, no. 2 (2006): 220, 221. https://www.medievalists.net/2016/01/the-influence-of-christianity-on-medicine-from-graeco-roman-times-up-to-the-renaissance/.

Smith, T., "The Knights of Saint John and the Hospitals of the Latin West," *Speculum* 3, no. 4 (1978): 709–733. https://www.journals.uchicago.edu/doi/epdf/10.2307/284 9782.

Snyder, Thomas L., "The Great Flu Crisis at Mare Island Navy Yard, and Vallejo, California," *Navy Medicine* 94, no. 5 (2003): 25–29.

Uyeki, Barbara T., Jernigan, D., and Tumpey, T., "Historical and Clinical Aspects of the 1918 H1N1 Pandemic in the United States," *Virology* 527 (2019): 32–37. https://www.sciencedirect.com/science/article/pii/S0042682218303313?via%3Dihub.

Unpublished Paper

Risse, G.B., "Medicalization: Hospitals Become Sites of Medical Care and Learning" (2004). https://www.academia.edu/10342059/Medicalization_Hospitals_Become_Site_of_Medical_Care_and_Learning.

Blog Posts

Snyder, T.L., "There's the Medical Corps and the Dental Corps and the...." (Part 3 of a five-part series on the Navy's nine "corps" of which five are medical), *Of Ships and Surgeons*, November 20, 2020. https://ofshipssurgeons.wordpress.com/2020/11/20/theres-the-medical-corps-and-the-dental-corps-and-the-part-3-of-a-5-part-series-on-the-navys-nine-corps-of-which-five-are-medical/.

Other Online Sources

Bay Area Radio Museum, Bay Area Radio Hall of Fame, "Timeline_KSFO." https://bayarearadio.org/history-index/timeline_ksfo.

Historic American Buildings Survey, National Park Service, Department of the Interior Washington, D.C. 20240 HABS No. CA-1543 HABS No. CP,-154.3 ADDENDUM TO: Mare Island Naval Shipyard, Mare Island Vallejo, Solano County, California. http://lcweb2.loc.gov/master/pnp/habshaer/ca/ca2500/ca2540/data/ca2540data.pdf.

Massachusetts Institute of Technology, "News of the Classes," *The Technology Review* 1872, vol. 23 (1921). https://books.google.com/books?id=hK0PAQAAIAAJ&pg= PA627&lpg=PA627&dq=ervin+s+hubbard+architect&source=bl&ots=EP7_fJf-4q&sig=dGxljeV57nTNWOZ7AQQVdvT_Wik&hl=en&sa=X&ved=0CDMQ6A EwCGoVChMI77yg3Yq0yAIVAT6ICh1uQQgn#v=onepage&q=ervin%20s%20 hubbard%20architect&f=false.

Bibliography

Metropolitan Transportation Commission—Association of Bay Area Governments, *Bay Area Census*, City of Vallejo, Decennial Census Data for the Years 1880–1940. http://www.bayareacensus.ca.gov/cities/Vallejo50.htm#1940.

Reference: "Asphaltum." https://books.google.com/books?id=Vs23AAAAIAAJ&pg PA291&lpg=PA291&dq=asphaltum+pipes&source=bl&ots=B1TXNAqqmV&sig= 2ncBeA6GGsC8Y50YJSOeQIKDla4&hl=en&sa=X&ved=0CCAQ6AEwAWoVCh MI87vI9bmiyAIVkpWICh296gp1#v=onepage&q=asphaltum pipes&f=false.

Reference: "Candela." http://en.wikipedia.org/wiki/Candela.

Reference: "Patent 226338." http://www.google.com/patents/US226338.

Savage-Smith, Emilie, *Islamic Culture and the Medical Arts* (Bethesda: National Library of Medicine, National Library of Medicine, 1994). An online version of a brochure to accompany an Exhibition in Celebration of the 900th Anniversary of the Oldest Arabic Medical Manuscript in the Collections of the National Library of Medicine, National Library of Medicine, Bethesda, Maryland. https://www.nlm.nih.gov/exhibition/islamic_medical/index.html#toc.

U.S. Department of Commerce, Bureau of the Census, *Historical Statistics of the United States, 1789–1945*, U.S. Government Printing Office, 1949, 300. http://www2.census.gov/prod2/statcomp/documents/HistoricalStatisticsoftheUnitedStates1789-1945.pdf.

Index

Numbers in ***bold italic*** indicate pages with illustrations

ambulance boats (Mare Island innovation) 135, ***136***

Baldwin, Elvira (first woman employee in hospital and Navy Yard) 66
Bates, Surg. Gen. Newton L. 59, 65
Berryhill, Thomas A. 126
Bishop, William S. 21, 23, 24, 25
"Brace Shop" (artificial limb shop) 154, 158, 159, 165
Bradley, George P. 85, 88, 89
Braisted, Surg. Gen. William C. 121, 128, 132, 135, 138
Brown, Calvin (Navy civil engineer, supervisor of construction) 26, 33, 34
Browne, John Mills 18, 29, 31, 33–40, 42, 43, 44, 49, 57, 58, 62, 66, 70, 71, 77
Browne, Surg. Gen. John Mills 48, 65, 80, 81, 82

Churchill, Winston ("Twice a Citizen" characterization of Reservists) 1, 179 *preface n* 1
Clifton, Alfred L. 151, 152
closure, plans for 150, 163, 164, 166, 167, 168, 169, 170, 171, 172, 173
Colhoun, CDRE E.R. 62
Combat Systems Technical Schools Command (successor to hospital) 175
Craven, CDRE Thomas T. 29
creativity and resourcefulness in California 2

Dahlberg, Andrew (contractor) 88, 89
Daily Alta California (newspaper) 32, 69
Dungan, J.S. 49, 50, 61, 67, 68, 77

earthquake 33, 34, 82–86, 111, 112

Farenholt, Ammen 126–134, 136
Farragut, Commander David (founder of Mare Island Naval Ship Yard) 17, 41
Foltz, Surg. Gen. Jonathan M. 49

Gates, Manley F. 120, 121
Gihon, Albert L. 47, 59, 65, 73, 74, 75, 78, 79
Goldsborough, CDRE John R. 38, 39
granary ("Temporary Hospital") 21, 24, ***25***
Grapevine (Mare Island Navy Yard newspaper) 158, 159, 160, 161
Great White Fleet 114
Grier, Surg. Gen. William 71
Gunnell, Surg. Gen. Francis M. 73, 74

Hawke, James A. 93, 94, 95, 96, 97, 98, 99, 100
Hogan, Bartholomew 164
Holman, Charles J. 155
Holman, Emile (Stanford professor, Navy Reservist) 152–153
Hope, Bob (entertainer) 161
Horowitz, Bureau Chief Phineas T. 28, 29, 30, 31, 33
Hospital Corps (enlisted) 93–95
Hudson, Adrian 47, 48, 55

Imola Annex (psychiatric, at Napa State Hospital) 156
USS *Independence* 20, 21, ***23***, 57, 180 *Chap 1 n* 2
infection 60, 99, 104, ***105***, 109, 110, 112, 113; new contagious building 153
influenza ("Spanish Flu") 127–132; cartoon ***129***; holiday decorations ***131***
intrepid men and women 2

Jordan, Dennis (San Francisco contractor) 32, 33, 34, 35, 89

207

Index

Kessler, Henry Howard (rehabilitation specialist, director of the Brace Shop) 159
Kindleberger, Charles P. 139, 140
Kirkland, RAdm. W.A. 83, 84
Kyser, Kay (bandleader) 161

laboratory (hospital) 113, 114, 129, 133, *134*
legal tender notes (Civil War currency) 24
Lemmon, Sue (Navy Yard historian) 66, 67
library, medical (hospital) 76
Lovering, Phillips A. 120

Mare Island Bulletin (newspaper) 129
McArthur, John, Jr. (architect) 28, 29, 30
McDougal, Capt. D.W. 29
McIntire, Surg. Gen. Ross T. 147, 150, 151, 152, 156, 160,
Messersmith, John S. 20
Miller, RAdm. M. 94
Mitchell, B. Reusch 18
Murphy, Charles (Vallejo contractor) 33; 50
Murphy, Joseph A. 143, 144

Naval Hospital, Mare Island: original *41*, 42; replacement 86–92, *91*
Neilson, John L. 146
nurses (female) 115, **116**, 116, 117, 118

Oakland, California, U.S. Naval Hospital 150, 159, 164, 168, 169, 170, 171
Osler, William (Johns Hopkins Professor of Medicine) 77
Outpatient Clinic (Navy/Department of Veterans Affairs) 175, *175*
Owen, John P. 154

Peck, George 51, 52, 53, 63, 64, 71, 72, 73
Perry, Wendell H. 163
Persons, Remus C. 112, 113, 114, 117
Poindexter, William M. 86
psychiatry (alienist, PTSD) 109, 138, 155–158; hospital *139*

recreation (Red Cross) building 134, *135*
Reservists, Naval (called up for service) 148, 150, 151, 152
residences (hospital executive officer, and chief surgeon) 77–82, *82*, 98–103, *102*, 107
Riggs, Surg. Gen. Charles E. 144

Rixey, Surg. Gen. Presley M. 101, 102, 103, 104, 105, 108, 109, 114, 115, 117
Robinson, Somerset 45, 46, 54, 55
Russell, CDRE John Henry 54
Russian Squadron 69, 70

Sacramento Daily Union (newspaper) 82
San Francisco (Morning) Call (newspaper) 82, 83, 88
San Pedro California News Pilot (newspaper) 140
Selfridge, Capt. Thomas Oliver 23, 24
Simons, Manly H. 103, 104, 106, 107, 108, 109, 116, 117, 118, 119
Sonoma Mission Inn (U.S. Naval Rest Center) 157
Stitt, Surg. Gen. Edward R. 137, 138, 139
Stoddart, David (contractor) 43, 44
Stokes, Surg. Gen. Charles F. 120
Suddards, James 61, 68, 76
Swanson, Surg. Gen. Clifford A. 164

theory of medical architecture 2
Toffelmier, Lt. Cmdr. Douglas D. (Reservist, orthopedic surgeon, founder of the Brace Shop) 158
Touro University California (current owner of hospital facilities) 2, 176
trainees 153
Tryon, Surg. Gen. James R. 94

vacuum cleaner (hospital) 120
Vallejo Evening Chronicle (newspaper) 42
Vallejo Times-Herald (newspaper) 142, 143, 145, 146
Van Reypen, Surg. Gen. William K. 55, 85, 86, 87, 94, 95, 97, 98

Wales, Surg. Gen. Phillip Skinner 51, 72
USS *Warren* 18, *19*
water (shortage and supply) 22, 33, 35, 36, 42–49, 74, 104
WAVES (Women Accepted for Volunteer Emergency Service) 153
Whelan, Bureau Chief William 20, 24
Wood, Surg. Gen. William Maxwell 36, 38
Woods, G.W. 44, 48, 49, 56, 59, 60, 65, 66, 67, 75, 82, 83

X-ray (for diagnosis) 25, 76, 113

.

www.ingramcontent.com/pod-product-compliance
Lightning Source LLC
Chambersburg PA
CBHW032043300426
44117CB00009B/1176